Dr. Kathryn Shafer's book, *Falling Awake: The FUN® Guide to Integrating EMDR, Brainspotting, and Yoga Nidra for Trauma and Self-Regulation*, is a remarkable and transformative work that bridges the worlds of trauma therapy and spiritual growth. I am deeply impressed by Dr. Shafer's ability to integrate EMDR, Brainspotting, and Yoga Nidra, providing a comprehensive approach to healing and self-regulation. Her book is a beacon of hope for those seeking profound healing and personal growth. Dr. Shafer's commitment to well-being and her ability to communicate complex concepts in an accessible manner make this a must-read for mental health professionals, trauma survivors, and seekers of self-knowledge alike.

Rachel Epstein, Esq., director, American Institute for Mental Imagery

* * *

Dr. Kathy Shafer's book, *Falling Awake*, is a compendium of clinical wisdom and healing stories that both inform and inspire. Dr. Shafer writes from the heart and the head, clearly passionate about the important, timely information she is conveying. As the founder and developer of Brainspotting, I can say that Dr. Shafer has done a wonderful job of conveying the foundation and nuance of Brainspotting theory and practice. This book is a must-read!

David Grand, PhD, psychotherapist, founder and author of Brainspotting: The Revolutionary New Therapy for Rapid and Effective Change

* * *

Kathryn Shafer's book emphasizes the most important, often missed, neurological components of psychotherapy by introducing readers to several important and diverse therapies that stimulate and/or calm different parts of the brain. I recommend this book to anyone searching for ways to help clients or themselves to become calm, mindful, trauma-free, and present.

Robin Shapiro, LICSW, psychotherapist, clinical consultant, writer, lecturer

* * *

Dr. Kathryn Shafer is passionate about teaching the brainbody connection for optimal functioning. A book filled with fascinating and empowering information that educates and inspires all on a journey of healing and transformation.

Grace Van Berkum, R.H.N.

* * *

Dr. Kathy Shafer is a consummate clinician who is well-versed in the therapies she describes here. I am fortunate to know her from her work in Brainspotting therapy and greatly appreciate her attunement to clients, which is key no matter what type of therapy one utilizes.

You will get a wonderful feel for what each method she describes holds from the way Dr. Shafer writes of these therapies about which she is passionate and knowledgeable. She has an engaging sense of humor that makes some of the more detailed concepts easy to understand and digest.

As a Brainspotting Trainer, I hope you may be moved to train in one of these therapies to enhance what you already do so well. You will be richer for it and gain some wonderful new tools that work at a deep brainbody level to benefit your clients.

Deb Antinori, MA, LPC, FT, RDT, Brainspotting senior trainer

* * *

A "fun" combination of treatment approach history, user-friendly techniques, case examples, and self-disclosure.

Roy Kiessling, LISW, founder/CEO, EMDR Consulting

* * *

Helping people to have FUN® in their trauma recovery journey is what Kathy shares through her extensive education, trainings, self-care, self-practice, and client experiences. This book, an introduction to complementary practices, is filled with exercises and case examples for the reader, especially a trained therapist, on how integrating several evidence-based treatment modalities and knowing what techniques might be teamed together can assist the therapist to help someone fall but continue to remain awake and alert during their treatment, especially with trauma.

Susan Tebb, PhD, LSW, RYT-500, MSW, C-IAYT, professor emerita, vice president of the Board for the International Association of Yoga Therapists

* * *

Refresh your clinical practice and have more fun in the treatment room! There is much richness in *Falling Awake* for mental health professionals: how Dr. Shafer's FUN® Program "brainbody" practices are applied in compassionate ways to empower the clients to establish goals and reach them; how EMDR can unlink those "touchstone" events in our lives to free us from emotional repetition; how Brainspotting works on a subcortical level to release emotional blocks without the need for words; how Yoga Nidra and other therapeutic yoga interventions can restore emotional balance; how to match the therapeutic intervention with the client's needs; and how the modalities might be integrated for the client's healing. But the true gifts of *Falling Awake* are the case stories, which moved this reader to tears more than once. Dr. Schafer knows when a personal sharing might be what the client needs to move forward in their healing, and she shows us how and when to combine EMDR or Brainspotting with Yoga Nidra. *Falling Awake* will give you the confidence to integrate the "brainbody" practices into your own healing work with clients and expand your self-care toolbox.

Amy Weintraub, MFA, E-RYT 500, C-IAYT, YACEP, founder of the LifeForce Yoga® Healing Institute and author of Yoga Skills for Therapists

* * *

Falling Awake stands as a testament to the many years of study, work, and dedication that Dr. Kathryn Shafer has brought to the field of healing. This book is friendly and fun—Dr. Kathy shares her passion generously, allowing the reader to gain integrative knowledge of some of the more recent and highly effective therapies on offer. It is such a valuable resource for anyone evaluating what therapy to make use of personally or study professionally. I love Dr. Kathy's honoring of fun and playfulness as part of the process of coming to wholeness. I honor and recognize that as she has undertaken the serious work of tackling society's tough issues through her community involvement, she has kept balance in her own life through music, movement, deep self-care, and good company. That shines through in this book. Today is the day to read this book and bring some FUN into your life!

Durga Leela, author of Yoga of Recovery: Integrating Yoga and Ayurveda with Modern Recovery Tools for Addiction

Falling Awake

of related interest

Yoga on Prescription
The Yoga4Health Social Prescribing Protocol
Paul Fox and Heather Mason
Foreword by Sat Bir Singh Khalsa
ISBN 978 1 78775 975 6
eISBN 978 1 78775 976 3

Trauma-Informed and Trauma-Responsive Yoga Teaching
A Universal Practice
Catherine Cook-Cottone and Joanne Spence
Forewords by Dr. Shirley Telles and Dr. Gail Parker
ISBN 978 1 83997 816 6
eISBN 978 1 83997 817 3

Sensory-Enhanced Yoga® for Self-Regulation and Trauma Healing
Lynn Stoller
Forewords by Stephen Cope and Joseph Le Page
ISBN 978 1 91208 513 2
eISBN 978 1 91208 514 9

FALLING AWAKE

The FUN® Guide to Integrating EMDR, Brainspotting, and Yoga Nidra for Trauma and Self-Regulation

Kathryn Shafer, PhD

Foreword by Kamini Desai, PhD

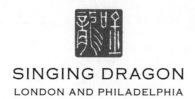

SINGING DRAGON
LONDON AND PHILADELPHIA

First published in Great Britain in 2025 by Singing Dragon,
an imprint of Jessica Kingsley Publishers
Part of John Murray Press

2

A CIP catalogue record for this title is available from the
British Library and the Library of Congress

ISBN 978 1 83997 789 3
eISBN 978 1 83997 790 9

Printed and bound in Great Britain by CPI Group

Jessica Kingsley Publishers' policy is to use papers that are natural,
renewable and recyclable products and made from wood grown in
sustainable forests. The logging and manufacturing processes are expected
to conform to the environmental regulations of the country of origin.

Singing Dragon
Carmelite House
50 Victoria Embankment
London EC4Y 0DZ

www.singingdragon.com

John Murray Press
Part of Hodder & Stoughton Limited
An Hachette UK Company

The authorised representative in the EEA is Hachette Ireland, 8 Castlecourt Centre,
Castleknock Road, Castleknock, Dublin 15, D15 YF6A, Ireland

Dedicated to: Den Den, Bentley, Jerry, Robin, David, Deb, Sheri, Chrissy, Kamini, Carolyn, Roy, Sue, Shay, Carlene, Grace, and most of all Patty—who are my tribe, hold the fort, and keep the porch light on... Go Tigers!

God, Goddess, Universe, Higher Power, grant me the serenity to accept the people I cannot change, the courage to change the one I can, and the wisdom to know that one is me...

ADULT CHILDREN OF ALCOHOLICS SERENITY PRAYER, REVISED BY KATHRYN SHAFER FROM THE 12-STEP PROGRAM 'ADULT CHILDREN OF ALCOHOLICS AND DYSFUNCTIONAL FAMILIES'

Contents

Foreword

Welcome to a journey of self-discovery, healing, and transformation. The pages of this book hold a wealth of wisdom and practical guidance for therapists, clinicians, and anyone interested in their own path to well-being. *Falling Awake: The FUN® Guide to Integrating EMDR, Brainspotting, and Yoga Nidra for Trauma and Self-Regulation* is more than just a guide; it is a roadmap to self-discovery and empowerment.

Dr. Kathryn Shafer introduces us to the fascinating realm of trauma neuroscience, unraveling the intricacies of the brainbody connection and unveiling the transformative potential of therapies like EMDR (Eye Movement Desensitization and Reprocessing), Brainspotting, and Yoga Nidra in promoting healing and self-regulation. *Falling Awake* stands as testament to the ever-evolving intersection of mental health and neuroscience. It delves profoundly into the mind–body connection, seamlessly weaving together science, mindfulness, and experiential therapies into a holistic approach.

In the realm of psychotherapy, it is now abundantly clear that the body's biochemistry shapes our state of mind just as our state of mind influences the body's biochemistry. At the core of this book lies a profound question: Do our beliefs give rise to our experiences, or do our experiences give rise to our beliefs? This question strikes at the heart of our perceptions, actions, and ultimately, our well-being.

Dr. Shafer's FUN® Program skillfully addresses this complex issue by employing a multifaceted approach. This innovative program is firmly grounded in the principles of cognitive behavioral therapy (CBT), offering a robust framework for challenging and reshaping erroneous beliefs. Simultaneously, it incorporates cutting-edge brainbody techniques that can play a pivotal role in fostering a physiological environment conducive to acquiring essential skills such as self-observation, conscious decision-making and the development of a resilient nervous system capable of maintaining composure in situations that would typically trigger reactivity.

While conventional approaches have traditionally operated from a "top-down," thought-centric model, Dr. Shafer presents us with integrated brainbody alternatives for those for whom talk therapy alone may not be the most effective path. She illuminates how the introduction of specific brainbody experiences can shift our perceptions and beliefs. What sets this book apart is Dr. Shafer's emphasis on self-empowerment. She urges readers to become the architects of their own well-being, embarking on their own unique healing journey. As she astutely notes, there is no one-size-fits-all approach to healing, and each individual's path is distinct.

Whether you are a therapist, a clinician or an individual seeking self-improvement, the value of this book is immeasurable. Dr. Shafer is a seasoned clinician with extensive knowledge and experience derived from years of study and exploration with her clients. She offers not just a foundational understanding of these techniques, but also practical, step-by-step guidance, exercises, and scripts that you can apply to yourself and share with your clients.

Dr. Shafer guides us through this intricate landscape with enthusiasm, clarity, and compassion. She reminds us that healing is not just about symptom relief but also about understanding the deeper causes of "dis-ease." It is about listening to the messages our bodies and minds are trying to convey and responding with kindness and curiosity (Bergner 2022).

These practices are not just techniques; they are gateways to understanding and harnessing the immense potential of our own mind–body connection. In these pages you will find the tools to become more self-aware, to navigate the challenges of life with resilience, and to tap into the profound wisdom of your own brainbody system. You will learn how to "fall awake," to pay attention to your thoughts and beliefs, and to embrace a path of self-care and self-regulation.

As someone who has devoted their life's work to a brainbody technique known as Yoga Nidra and who has written extensively on the subject, it is both refreshing and hopeful to witness the integration of Yoga Nidra and similar practices into the clinical setting, with Dr. Shafer as a pioneering figure in the field.

As you embark on this journey through the pages of *Falling Awake*, I encourage you to approach it with an open heart and an inquisitive mind. Explore the practices and techniques presented here, experiment with them, and discover what resonates with you and your clients. Remember that you have the power to shape each unique healing path, and this book is a valuable companion on that journey. May this book be a source of inspiration, healing, and growth on the path to wellness.

With warmest regards,

Kamini Desai, PhD
Author, Yoga Nidra: The Art of Transformational Sleep
Co-Founder, I AM Yoga Nidra
Founder and Director, I AM Education

Introduction

THE BODY KEEPS THE SCORE—AND THE BRAIN MAINTAINS A LEDGER

How many more trainings and certifications do I need? When is enough training or self-help enough? There are so many therapies and types of therapists...I don't have time to try them all! Seeking help is too expensive... Do you want to live?

Hey there! Now that I have your attention... Are you happy? Feeling stuck or overwhelmed? Are you ready to understand how your brain can help you "fall awake?" You must be since you have opted to pick up and read this book. As Dorothy herself found after she took the challenging journey down the yellow brick road to see the Wizard of Oz, she had the power herself the whole time—to accomplish her mission and go home—and so do you. You have the power within you to do anything you want. Pay attention to what you are thinking and saying to yourself as you read this book. The potential to change your life relies on you recognizing the power of your mind and what you believe: Do your beliefs create your experiences, or do your experiences create your beliefs? Stay tuned...as we are healing at the brain's pace.

This book is for therapists to use with clients as well as for those clinicians interested in starting or continuing on their own healing path. If you are new to therapy, self-care practices, or the "mindful healing arts," welcome. Or maybe you are curious about therapy, advanced therapy training, wanting to start but not sure what type of therapy to do or training to take—if so, this book is for you! And if you are a seasoned practitioner and seeker of self-care (Chödrön 2010, 2022; Chopich and Paul 1990), or just curious about other healing practices but wondering what to do next, or if what you are doing isn't helping, or you are getting bored or burned out, great!

There are more ways to find help and stay healthy in a "brainbody" way than ever before. Instead of the common reference to the "mindbody" or "wholebody healing," I refer to the "brainbody" because I am not sure the importance of the power of the brain (where beliefs originate) is always included in the healing process! The brain is the power center, like the central processing unit of a computer. As such, the brain records and stores everything (nothing is ever deleted permanently, which can happen when you hit the delete key on the computer). The brain tells the body how to respond to input it receives—hence the "brainbody."

Some ways are based on scientific evidence, neuroscience, and other data, while some self-help and psychotherapy practices remain "under scrutiny," or can challenge the Know It All or Skeptic in us. Whatever camp you may find yourself in, it doesn't matter because we all need to start somewhere—no matter what race, creed, color, sexual preference, or even how much money we have. And we can begin by just focusing on our breathing. Try it now: Breathe. Again, take a normal short inhale through the nose, followed by a loooooong exhale out through the mouth. Try this again a few times...gently. Now try experimenting with this: On your next gentle inhale say the word "let" (to yourself) and exhale the word "go" (you can do this with the eyes open or closed). Try this several times. Relax your shoulders, elbows, and hands. Notice the left foot...the right foot...

Pause for a moment and notice how you feel now. What are you sensing in the body? Has something shifted? Maybe you are calmer? Or has this made you more anxious? Just notice what happens when you focus on the breath... It's that simple. When we keep *thinking* about doing something to stop the thoughts or stories we keep telling ourselves, know that it will take time to change the beliefs we have created during our lifetime that are not serving us or that are keeping us "stuck."

In my private practice, clients often tell me that they feel as though they are "falling apart" (when they may actually be *falling awake*). Some also ask "What happened to me? How did I get into this mess/situation (again)?" Or they may come to the session with the belief, "Nothing is ever going to change. I have tried everything." When we start to explore and bring into *focus* the language that is being used to describe what is going on in their lives, or what they are thinking about and why, we can consider the question I just asked: "Do your beliefs create your experiences, or do your experiences create your beliefs?" I also ask, "What brought you to therapy *now*?" or "What do you want in your life *now*, to make things different?" In some cases, when things seem so bleak or hopeless, I may ask: "Do you want to live?" I am still asking these questions after all these years, as it is important to think about what we are saying to ourselves—as well as what details we haven't thought or talked about.

A client I'll call David, 58, who is self-employed and has been in therapy on and off his whole life, describes therapy like this:

> I have this truck. Let's say that it has 475,000 miles on it. It has lasted this far because of the care and maintenance I have given it. And because I am meticulous about this machine, why would I not apply the same philosophy to my physical and mental health? Just like a turbo charger or high-end vehicle, every so often I need a tune-up and a check-up under the hood too. To me therapy is like recharging the battery, filling up the fuel tank, and getting an oil change.

Since I wrote my first book in 2000 and decided to trademark The FUN® Program, a lot has happened to keep me challenging my thinking, asking more questions, and exploring new information. Here is some of what's gone on and been on my mind:

I met Dennis at Puffy's Tavern in New York City after running my third marathon (1999). Dennis has since become my life partner and was by my side when I was going through and survived stage 3 breast cancer.

We are seeing countries at war (Putin invading Ukraine), conditions being imposed on freedom of speech (Florida Governor DeSantis removing certain books from the educational curriculum), and women restricted from having choice over their body (the reversal of *Roe v. Wade*). There were also the terrorist attacks of 9/11 (2001), the Covid-19 pandemic (2020) (from which we are still feeling the impact), the attack on Capitol Hill in Washington, DC (2021), and an increase in gun violence.

More children are being shot in their schools, and mass shootings are happening more often than we would like to admit. We now recognize that Black Lives Matter, we recognize LGBTQ rights, we know about QAnon, we keep hearing how an election was stolen and how citizens of the United States are moving abroad because of politics and because of an increase in violence (Van Dam 2022).

The abuse of opiates has increased drastically, with new plant-based ceremonies and psychedelic psychotherapy (Ayahuasca, mushrooms, MDMA) getting a nod from the FDA. We have experienced devastating hurricanes, floods, fires, and temperatures spiking to unprecedented and dangerous heights.

The time is now more than ever to embrace self-regulation so we can all calm the f*** down! This is the essence of falling and remaining awake! We need to pay attention, and not fall asleep (stay tuned...).

In response to all this, what's on my mind these days (as well as on my clients' minds) are conversations about whether it's safe to go to public places since now we have Zoom, and more things are available online, making it more convenient than ever to stay indoors: shopping for everything, telehealth, virtual medical and psychotherapy appointments, attending school, webinars on-demand, even live conferences and workshops, and attempting to make in-person therapy sessions the rare exception rather than the norm! However, thanks to Zoom and virtual medical appointments, which became a necessity during Covid-19, we are now facing concerns about Artificial Intelligence attempting to replace the live, attuned presence of a trained professional responding to interactions with a client (Barker 2024). We don't have to be together anymore and co-regulate. (Huh? Chapter 1 is coming...)

And many people I admire, who have influenced my work as a clinician, have died: famous people—Betty White, Michael Jackson, David Bowie, Tom Petty, Prince, Whitney Houston, Amy Winehouse, Charlie Watts, Lou Reed, Tina Turner, Elizabeth II, Sinead O'Connor, Jimmy Buffet, Jeff Beck, and Suzanne Somers, to name just a few—as well as friends and family members, including my parents, Dr. Gerald Epstein (my mentor), my first Golden Retriever JJ, and others I care about who have passed since the publication of this book. And Lady Gaga, Madonna, and Beyoncé return to touring *huge* live stadium concerts as well as The Rolling Stones, who have just released *Hackney Diamonds*, their first studio album of original music since 2005.

When we think about all this, no wonder people are HALT (Hungry, Angry, Lonely, or Tired), short-tempered, ready to argue, die by suicide, shoot each other, overdose, take lots of medication, quit their jobs, refuse to go back to work, or just be nice! And they are also not talking to each other in the supermarket, at a coffee shop, or after a yoga class. The planet keeps getting warmer, our food is not so clean and pure, and we are spending more time inside, just sitting around eating mindlessly, watching television, not sure if we should shake hands, hug each other, or touch our faces anymore, or whether it is safe to go to a live concert or eat outside at a restaurant!

All of this is why I am more motivated than ever to continue my part in helping humanity. To do my part to contribute to making the world a calmer, kinder community, I decided to write this book and found a home for it with Singing Dragon publishers (according to Chinese astrology, 2024 is the Year of the Dragon (Dore 2021)). The time is *now* for all of us to embrace the power of imagination, just like John Lennon sang to us, and to "fall awake." To do this, we must first and foremost look at what is going on within ourselves, as this is where falling and remaining awake begins. Self-care must be a priority, and so this book provides a structure for tending to ourselves while having compassion and consideration for others.

It takes *focused* energy and self-discipline to be and remain awake, but the rewards are worth it. When we begin to pay attention to what we are thinking about (or imagining), and to the symptoms of what our complex emotions and physical illnesses are trying to tell us, we discover that they are significantly influenced by internal and external toxins, lifestyles, and circumstances, which become known to us as the beliefs we think and the behaviors we do. These factors, which are linked to the stressors mentioned, can result in the reactive emotional and behavioral responses and dysregulation in our nervous system.

In *Falling Awake: The FUN® Guide to Integrating EMDR, Brainspotting, and Yoga Nidra for Trauma and Self-Regulation*, psychotherapists, addiction counselors, yoga therapists, healing professionals, and other seekers will learn the following: the science behind what happens in the brain impacted by trauma, how trauma-informed practices can calm the brain down and heal it, an understanding of the value and limitations of talk therapy, how to employ The FUN® Program I developed, the timeless science of Yoga Nidra, and the neuroexperiential models of EMDR and Brainspotting. All these theoretically-diverse and evidence-based, trauma-informed practices can be easily integrated into different clinical settings. As a practical, hands-on introductory guidebook, *Falling Awake* offers therapists and their clients the explanation, mechanics, and proper application of these techniques to ethically and safely teach to themselves and their clients. While licensing, training, and seeking help from a certified professional is always recommended, the information and basics provided in this book will serve as a basic platform to begin your clinical and healing journey.

"Falling awake" is as natural as "paying attention," although we have many ways to stay distracted. Learning how to fall and remain awake, utilizing the wisdom of what I refer to as brainbody therapies (meaning wholebody therapies), will provide therapists and clients with specific cognitive-behavioral, mindful, mental imagery, and somatic psychology tools.

The benefits of integrating brainbody therapy tools into your practice can include:

- Motivation for clients to self-regulate.

- Increasing clients' feelings of self-competence and confidence as they understand the mechanics of the brainbody therapies.

- Empowering clients to embrace the control they have over themselves and their life circumstances from just paying attention to what they are thinking.

- Enhanced attunement in the therapeutic/helping/caring-for-you relationship.

Beginning with the end in mind—having fun on the healing journey—readers will learn the brainbody basics of mindful, self-regulation, integrating self-care practices, starting with The FUN® Program, a cognitive-behavioral approach to paying attention to what you are thinking and telling yourself about your life. I developed FUN® during my healing process after being hit by a drunk driver and used it extensively when I later faced (and recovered from) stage 3 breast cancer. The FUN® Program and brainbody wisdom practices that are offered in *Falling Awake* are all widely recognized and supported by neuroscience, psychology, mindfulness, experiential, and somatic therapies that have been revised and recognized by clinical research.

More importantly, FUN®, EMDR, Brainspotting, and Yoga Nidra are more than techniques to use when triggered between appointments; they can also be used as an integrated part of a person's life journey. The contents of this book provide a unique synergistic way of combining practices that are belief-driven, client-centered, within the scope of practice, and are specific to the presenting problem of the client: what they want or need—*now*.

Many of the licensed psychotherapists, addiction, and healing arts professionals whom I have trained, supervised, and worked with over the past 40 years are among the approximately 16 million Americans, and countless others internationally, who are currently exploring the benefits of, seeking information about, and training in, integrative mindfulness and brainbody approaches for emotional and physical health. These clinicians have become aware of the shifts in mood, release of complex emotions, and relief from psychological and physical pain such tools can provide in-and outside of the healthcare setting or yoga studio. What clients report and notice after a brainbody therapy session is that they feel more confident and hopeful when they experience the ability to control dysregulation, accompanied by changes in action and behavior.

What inspires the licensed clinicians and other health professionals who consult with me to try the brainbody therapies is that these simple tools create quicker changes than talk therapy alone can offer! The FUN® Program and techniques presented in this book create the possibility to make an amazing turn towards health. After much pain and frustration and time, children as young as six to people in their senior years have been inspired to assume a de-victimized stance by using a repertoire of simple tools for creating a better quality of life. Benefits enjoyed by those who use this program include significant relief from physical symptoms, freedom from old habits and limited thinking, higher energy levels, overall health improvement, and finding new ways to experience joy in living.

The explosion of interest and research in integrative and alternative practices and brainbody science has generated a new model of healing, one that encourages taking responsibility for our own well-being and fosters a curiosity to consider what else we can do differently to address our current life challenges. Being healthy means more than freedom from symptoms of "dis-ease." It means whole brainbody health. The FUN® approach to healing is different from a checking-the-boxes, medical viewpoint that focuses on what's "wrong," and then tries to "fix" it as fast as possible. While focusing on and removing physical symptoms provides relief from the immediate problem, this may only be temporary, leaving the deeper causes of dis-ease unexplored and likely to re-emerge.

There is now comparative clinical evidence that the psychotherapeutic techniques used in EMDR, Brainspotting, and body scan meditation (such as Yoga Nidra) for distressing memories and trauma, along with the deep connection between the client and therapist, are gaining respect and recognition in terms of efficacy (D'Antoni *et al.* 2022). Healing and sustained recovery involves examining the whole brainbody—the attuned, present awareness process between the distraught/stressed-out/anxious client and the attentive regulated therapist, a process that is accomplished organically, affectively, and somatically during the session by turning inward and *toward* the dis-ease while listening, nonjudgmentally, to what this annoying or scary "visitor" is trying to tell us (the cancer, depression, accident, suicide, anxiety, grief, guilt…). In other words, can our client's nervous system trust that we (the clinician, yoga therapist, etc.) are a predictable, reliable, consistent caring presence that wants to nonjudgmentally help them?

For prospective clients and clinicians/therapists, it is important to take the time to access and allow the "problem," "symptoms," or "issue" to "speak." In other words, what emotions, memories, beliefs, or "stories" need to be discussed and addressed for healing and relief (symptom reduction) to happen? Listening to what information the current symptom or problem behavior is giving can serve as a compass or guide. This can be the shining star that leads you toward a place within yourself that holds the information, knowledge, and wisdom for creating an effective recovery plan and beginning to live disease-free. I encourage you to use The FUN® Program and to try the brain-based wisdom approaches for healing included in this book (EMDR, Brainspotting, and Yoga Nidra). You may decide to see a trained, certified, and licensed healing arts professional or not. Remember—you cannot do it alone, but you must try something different (if your way is not working).

It can take as little as 21 days to change a habit and establish a baseline to begin the healing journey. Once a change in habits and beliefs begins, this healing/recovery/remission becomes fulfilling in ways that go far beyond the original problem or diagnosis. Relationships, energy, and productivity are affected. Anxiety, anger, fatigue, despair, resentment, and irritability are modified as well. And when you make the FUN® approach part of your everyday life, the transformation remains lasting and powerful. Remember—what you practice, you strengthen—and this is when a shift happens.

The message of this book is simple: It urges you to become your own authority and teacher. It also shows you there is more than one way to create your healing goals. Talk therapy may or may not be part of your journey as well as the brainbody therapies discussed here. Please remember that your behavioral health goals may be accomplished faster and easier with the help of a trained professional and/or support group (12-step and otherwise). For example, researchers showed promising long-term results (after a six-month follow-up) comparing the interventions of cognitive behavioral therapy (CBT) and yoga with older adults presenting difficulty with insomnia, worry, and anxiety (Whitlock Burton 2022). While there were no significant differences between the two interventions, the important implication of the study was for informed clinicians and healthcare providers to tell their clients *the choice is up to you, and trying either one of these (or both) is probably going to help.*

No disease process, prognosis, or treatment plan is carved in stone; neither is the way you choose to address it. This is not to say that you should throw away your medications and disregard your doctor's advice. However, what is strongly suggested here is that there is no right or wrong way to address what is upsetting you, only *your own way*. And this involves your willingness not to deny, dismiss, or omit what is going on with your behavior (including alcohol and drug misuse), emotions, triggers, or physical symptoms, and to instead pay attention and take time to be honest about choices. Notice when you are judging yourself while on the journey to freedom from dis-ease. This is all part of falling awake.

How you can benefit from this book

Many people may find The FUN® Program useful and want to dig deeper but without talking so much (you may even want to become a FUN® therapist yourself). This is what the alternative brainbody approaches of EMDR, Brainspotting, and Yoga Nidra offer adults, teens, family members, curious seekers, and healthcare professionals. There are suggested setups, guidelines, gadgets, and pointers that practitioners learning and utilizing these treatment modalities often use. That said, through research and experience, we have also come to understand and trust that the brainbody knows exactly where to go and what to process when included and accessed in session. This healing or shift in awareness and behavior can occur with or without these props and "protocols" for the different issues or behavioral concerns that bring clients to the healing arts.

What I discuss in this book is how The FUN® Program and brainbody practices were created. I also talk about why and how the props and "setups" are used as guides during the different phases of the clinical session. I trust that you will then decide what additional training and practice guidelines to follow to keep you and your clients safe, and that you will adhere to the ethical guidelines of your profession. Please remember to first try anything in this book that is new to you, or that you have not done for yourself, before using it with a client.

For those interested in these practices (if you want to become a FUN®

trauma-informed therapist), I recommend that you find an experienced, trained, and perhaps licensed or certified practitioner to guide you. While none of the practices replaces what medication a doctor is prescribing or the guidance you are seeking from other healthcare professionals, once you understand and have used these practices often, there is less need to rely on the medical system as the complete authority over your own well-being. Instead, you will discover that you have options, and that you can develop new skills and behaviors to keep you feeling healthy, peaceful, and prosperous.

The toolbox of adaptable strategies provided here is pulled from my research, study, training, clinical experience, personal journey, and certification in multiple clinical methods, traditions, and lineages. They are guidelines for falling—and stay-ing—awake. I invite you to get curious and experiment with them. Sometimes one way works for a while, and then we need to shake it up and let the snow in the snow globe settle and go in a different direction.

How to use this book

Just as there is no "one" way to heal from trauma, addiction, betrayal, family dysfunc-tion, stress, and pain that occurs with dis-ease, there is no "right" way to read this book. How you approach the material presented here will reflect your own particular style of interest and learning. Some of you might enjoy reading through it slowly and deliberately. Others might skim through, and then choose to focus on a single method. You may prefer doing the exercises as they come up, or you may find you want to return to the techniques and exercises after you have an overall feel for each method and have Googled it (yes, you will want to check it out with "the authority" known as the World Wide Web). You may enjoy underlining passages that interest you or writing notes in the margins as you go along. You may also want to concentrate on something that attracts your attention and stay there for a while before moving on. Whether it takes you three weeks or three months, you will get the most out of this book by reading it at your own natural pace and exploring it all in your own way.

So! Are you ready to calm the f*** down, "fall awake," and have FUN® during the process? If so, read on, put on your seat belts, take off your blinders, stay curious about your reactions (no judgment), lie down, and go with that...all will be revealed when we stop and let go...

CHAPTER 1

Brain Basics—Prepare to Encounter Your Mind...

> *Do your beliefs create your experiences, or do your experiences create your beliefs? (Dr. Gerald Epstein, personal communication)*
>
> *You are already divine. All you have to do is become human. (Swami Rama, quoted in Tigunait 2001, p.81)*

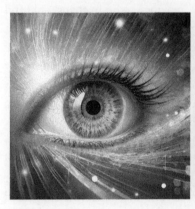 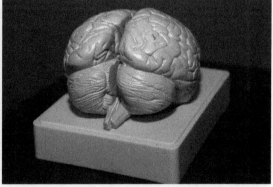

Hello and welcome to the brain! You are about to enter a vast world of neurodiversity—which I refer to as the "brain forest"—where every path is constantly adapting, maturing, and working together with the whole body to help you get out of danger, self-regulate, and stay healthy (Menon 2022). The world of mental health is in an extraordinary period of conceptual transformation. Research, integrating science from a variety of disciplines, is creating a multifaceted view of mental health that includes understanding how our brain and physical body are influenced by our beliefs, life experiences, and interpersonal relationships. Building on this concept of the brain forest, we need to include how an individual's health is impacted by the many aspects of the human experience. The heart of our well-being, according to Siegel (Siegel and Drulis 2023), includes understanding a concept called "interpersonal neurobiology:"

our brain's ability to adapt and learn, relying on the complex interaction and inter-connectedness of the personal, social, and natural environments in which we live.

Think of the brain as a forest you are going to wander into and explore. As your guide in this brain forest, I am taking you on a beginner's journey. Please know that I am neither a neuroscientist nor a brain expert; I am sharing with you the knowl-edge, training, and learning gained from experts in the field and from my work using these practices with my clients during my four-decade career as a psychotherapist, trauma and addiction professional, and yoga therapist. As such, I have continued my education and research, exploring exactly what role the brain and physical body play in the healing and personal growth processes. This became part of my passion for writing this book. The question that Dr. Gerald Epstein once asked me has fueled much of my fascination and study: Do your beliefs create your experiences, or do your experiences create your beliefs?

Contrary to what many of us were taught (if we were taught anything about the brain at all), we now know that the brain and the body (referred to from now on as the "brainbody") are not "hardwired" or designed to perform specific, unchanging tasks. Due to groundbreaking neuroscientific research, we have plausible neurophysiological explanations for the experiences described by those impacted by trauma. We know the brainbody "retunes" and adapts in response to threats in order to "feel safe" and "self-regulate" (Porges 2017, 2022). This concept of the brain's malleability means that the brainbody can reorganize itself throughout life, making the brain changeable and modifiable at any age. While we may think our brains are in charge, however, the heart of our daily experience and the way we navigate the world includes our understanding of the autonomic nervous system—our physical body (Dana 2021). Understanding how thinking, learning, and behaving turns our neural pathways on or off, thus shaping our brain anatomy, including our genes and activities of daily living (ADLs), may be among the most extraordinary discoveries of the twenty-first century (Doidge 2007).

The therapies addressed in this book—The FUN® Program, Eye Movement Desensitization and Reprocessing (EMDR), Brainspotting, and Yoga Nidra—all have similar but distinct methods of accessing these systems in the brainbody for expression, self-regulation, and continued growth and recovery, and all are supported by unique but similar neurological science to describe how and what happens when used in the psychotherapy session.

The aim of this chapter is to highlight and briefly present the evolving information and the importance of understanding what currently seem to be "the basics" of the complex workings of the brain for trauma and self-regulation. Please know that the science and facts about the brain as I present them are how I understand it. I am not a neurologist or brain expert, just a seeker (there's that word again), making sense of how I understand the functions of the brain. Note the information provided in this chapter, take what makes sense and is useful to you, leave the rest, and keep reading and discovering more about the brain forest! You can even completely forget about it if you are not interested! Just know that by starting to read this chapter, you are already "falling awake!"

Be prepared for what's happening in your brainbody!

First and foremost, according to Kase (2023) we cannot separate the biology (or the brain) from the person: "Despite the advances in psychology, psychotherapists (still) remain one of the few groups in the medical community that do not look at the organ they treat" (2023, p.2)—meaning the nervous system, which includes the brain and the body. "Neuro-informed counselling," Kase says, "recognizes that dysregulation and dysfunction in the nervous system leads to common clinical complaints like depression, anxiety, addiction, suicidality, personality disorders, and psychosis" (2023, p.3). Kase says that when we get curious about these symptoms, it often reveals the interventions needed to make the body heal. This neuro-informed approach shifts our clinical focus from pathologizing the dysfunction toward curiosity for the function of the dysfunction—exploring the meaning of the behavior versus becoming the label or diagnosis... "My anxiety," "My ADHD," "My cancer."

Are you beginning to see why understanding the mechanics of the brain is so important? Let's take a closer look under the hood (the skull), bypass the cerebral cortex (the cortical brain), and take the staircase that goes down into the basement of the brain (subcortical brain, limbic brain, and the brainstem). To become a brain-savvy being (Badenoch 2008, 2011, 2018), there are some key areas of the brain to understand: the prefrontal cortex (neocortex), the subcortical brain, the limbic system, and the brainstem. And just of note, the two major systems that the brain is involved with activating and regulating are: (1) the central nervous system, which consists of the brain, spinal cord, and all the nerves within our body, and (2) the autonomic nervous system, which is the part of the central nervous system that regulates involuntary body functions (breathing, heart rate, blinking eyes, etc.).

While we often refer to these as separate "sections" or "regions" of the brain, they function simultaneously and rely on each other for input to respond. Modern neuroscience research says that triune brain theory, referred to as the "three-part brain" (neocortex, limbic system, and basal ganglia), no longer accurately explains how the brain functions in everyday life or during a stressful or traumatic incident (Steffen, Hedges, and Matheson 2022).

According to Barrett (2021) we have just one brain, not three. Plato attempted to explain how the brain evolved with three layers, one for surviving, one for feeling, and one for thinking. This, according to Barrett, is how the triune brain theory developed, and "is one of the most successful and widespread errors of all science" (2021, p.15). Barrett continues, "You have one brain, not three. Move past Plato's ancient battle, we might need to fundamentally rethink what it means to be rational, what it means to be upset, what it means to be responsible for our actions, and perhaps what it means to be human" (2021, p.28).

Now let's visit the prefrontal cortex. The logical left part of your "upstairs brain" (checking out the facts of the situation, putting things in order, trying to understand and figure things out) is wondering what this chapter is going to teach you about the brain and why this is so important in the therapy session (Siegel and Payne Bryson 2015). You may even be thinking that you want to skip this chapter and move on to something else, like what you are going to have for dinner. At the same time, the right side of the "upstairs brain" (feelings, emotional information, creativity, autobiographical information) may be thinking that the information might be too overwhelming or not that important, and that you and/or your clients just want to know what "to do to feel better" or what is going to happen in the therapy session. Guess what? This means that right now, in this moment, the *whole brain and body* are involved in the falling awake process.

According to Carr (2023), nearly three decades after leaving Harvard, Dr. Bessel van der Kolk is currently the world's most famous living psychiatrist and author of the landmark trauma book *The Body Keeps the Score: Brain, Mind, and Body in the Healing of Trauma* (2014), which has spent 278 weeks and counting on *The New York Times* paperback nonfiction bestseller list (Doidge 2007, 2016). His claim to fame is his theory that trauma is a literal assault of the past into the present, which can produce physiological effects whether or not the traumatized person consciously remembers this event. Even after the trauma is "over," van der Kolk (2002) maintains that the body stays on alert, reliving the threat as if it is still happening *now*. While the body may keep the score, referring to the ways trauma is stored in the physical body, the brain (which is part of our body) maintains a ledger, and is also recording *everything*. You, like me, may be wondering why there is suddenly so much interest, emphasis, training, and publications in the mental health world about how the brain processes information—especially in the treatment of trauma or in times of just plain stress. It is because we are now finally acknowledging that everything we say, think, eat, and do impacts and involves the whole body, which includes the brain. I think we forget this sometimes.

Now awake and paying attention, you may be curious (a Dr. David Grand Brainspotting term—stay tuned) about what you are learning and thinking. You may be noticing physical sensations (an EMDR term—stay tuned), such as furrowing your eyebrows, yawning, running your hands through your hair, wanting to do your nails, get on your phone, or check your emails. Or you may be having emotions just reading about the brain. Whatever you are experiencing right now, your whole body (a Yoga Nidra phrase—stay tuned), including your brain, is involved.

Intense memories and thoughts may be real but are not true *now*

During challenging times, it is common for someone to say: "I feel like I am losing my mind" or "I just don't feel like myself, I have no energy" or "My mind is made up, I am fine" or even better, "I've been doing this for so long, nothing is going to change the way I think." Can you relate? I can.

The effects of life experiences and statements like these (also known as mind chatter or thinking in cognitive behavioral therapy (CBT), and the Monkey Mind in yoga) become attached and connected in complex ways to thousands of neural networks in the adaptive information processing (AIP model, an EMDR term) center of the brain. Therefore, the complex emotions and memories released and shared in the therapy session are real but *not true now* from a brain-based perspective. Huh?

Daily stressful events (the news, politics, violence, etc.), developmental situations (such as childhood sexual abuse, bullying, or identifying as LGBTQ), generational trauma (such as being from a BIPOC or Indigenous community), and other challenging realities (racism, sexism, antisemitism, domestic violence, corporate mobbing, to name just a few) affect each of us in diverse and unique ways, both overtly and covertly. The impact of how we respond to these life events is physically, emotionally, and neurologically different for each person. According to internationally renowned neuroscience researcher Dr. Damir Del Monte (2023), our brain is a very vulnerable organ, and all our psychosocial (life) experiences become "structures" that are stored in the brain. He says these "structures" are encoded in the brain and subsequently become expressed as "my experience," which, over time, becomes a belief or "story" about what happened at that place and time. It is this "my experience" that becomes hard-wired in the brain and eventually evolves into the intense feelings and memories that feel very real in the moment (negative cognition/beliefs—more EMDR terms!). Del Monte says all these structures become "my life and my experience" and are stored in the brain as "me" (aka "my" beliefs). And we can become very attached to these!

How these "structures" are expressed emotionally and behaviorally in the therapy session, in relationships, in cultures, and in family dynamics, seems to depend on a variety of factors such as when, where, and how long ago this event or situation happened, over what period of time (a one-time occurrence, or for many years or generations), and what coping strategies and supports were in place at the time (or not). All these structures seem to cluster and light up neural networks in addition to the amygdala (the fight, flight, freeze, or faint assessor), impacting at least 50 other places in the brain—all at the same time. Del Monte (2023) states that the brain is always working and sometimes gets expressed by a body ache (headache, stiff shoulders, back pain, etc.) that he refers to as the somatosensory nucleus. This, he says, makes the brain a sort of "sensory gate;" like an orchestra playing music in which every instrument is needed to create the sound we want to hear and directing us to what needs an adjustment or "tune up."

Referring to the neuroplasticity of the brain being vulnerable to outside influences, including the ability to be rigid, on alert, as well as flexible, revisits Dr. Epstein's question—Do our beliefs create our experiences, or do our experiences create our beliefs? Inquiring about and exploring this question helps us become "neuroplasticians"—students and practitioners of this evolving brainbody science. When clients come to therapy or seek help from the provider they have chosen, they show up describing disturbing experiences, often while releasing intense emotions. These acute reactions and physical feelings are "sensed" somatically and are stored in the subcortical brain closet, which leads to the spinal cord and travels down into the body (Doidge 2007). These are the areas involved in regulation where "the body keeps the score" and the mind "maintains a ledger" that cannot be accessed by talk therapy alone.

What "works" in the therapy session to access these deeper regions of the brain depends on a variety of factors—not only on what happened to the client, but also how you provide them with a secure, nonjudgmental, confidential space to be vulnerable so they can tell their story. This is called the therapeutic alliance and attunement (EMDR and Brainspotting terms!). We professionals must be able to hold a consistent, reliable, steady place for clients to "freak out," cry, scream, yell, and tell "my experience" in a confidential secure place while embracing the uncertainty of expression (a Dr. Grand Brainspotting term—coming up!), without engaging the cortical talking brain by asking questions and getting involved in the details. The brainbody session is where anything can happen, and all forms of expression are welcome. "Random" thoughts and "out of the blue" memories accessed may not make "sense" but are revealed so that the complex neural network of the subcortical brain can self-regulate, heal, and calmly let the cortical brain determine what is going on. In other words, a psychological shift cannot happen without a neurological one. Welcome to brain basics 101!

Making connections

In recent years, there has been a paradigm shift in understanding the unique presentations of physical complaints and "mental" disorders in behavioral health and primary care medicine. How we or our clients describe the "presenting problems" and what gets us to the healthcare providers we turn to depends on individual unique circumstances. What psychology, neuroscience, and behavioral health experts are now recognizing is that words have power—what we say to ourselves and to others matters and can influence the type of care we find and are provided with. Grounded in decades of both brain science and empirical clinical research, trauma-informed therapies are now attempting to bridge the gap between neuroscience, biology, psychiatry, and clinical practice. Infused with the impact of generational trauma, culture, race, sexual identity, and social media, we now know there is much more going on in the therapy session than what we can "see" or gather in contemporary client history taking.

The various interconnected regions of the brain are impacted by events from the beginning of the seventh month of fetal life (Merzenich 2013) and throughout the life span. To experience life in its fullness we need to experience childhood, become a teenager, then an adult, grow old, and learn from these stages or "parts" of our lives. According to Siegel and Payne Bryson (2015), the ability to control impulses, calm big feelings, and make good decisions ranks high on the list of feeling confident about ourselves. Since the area of the brain that regulates and controls these functions is not fully developed until our mid-twenties, what we were taught, when we were taught, and whether we understood what we were taught about self-regulation and communication from birth to adulthood influences how we think and behave. These early memories, stages of life, and daily life stressors are expressed emotionally and behaviorally in every clinical session. The Adverse Childhood Experiences Questionnaire (ACE-Q) (Felitti *et al*. 1998) and the Impact of Events Scale (IES) (Horowitz, Wilner, and Alvarez 1979) help us as professionals, and our clients, understand why the whole brainbody is responding the way it is, and that it stores this information.

Further research into the brainbody connection pertains to the role of the vagus nerve in emotion regulation, social connection, and the fear response. Polyvagal Theory (PVT), developed in 1994 by Dr. Stephen Porges (Porges, Doussard-Roosevelt, and Mait 1994), is the science of feeling safe (Kase 2023). PVT is a theoretical model, not a specific therapy; it is another way to understand how the brain responds to outside stimuli. Neuroception, as defined by Porges, is the body's home surveillance system. It is a function of the autonomic nervous system, which scans the environment for cues of safety and danger. According to Dana (2018), the autonomic nervous system's job is to survive in times of danger (fight, flight, freeze, or faint) and thrive in times of safety. According to Porges (2022) the vagus nerve (and the dorsal brake) plays a significant role in feeling safe and protection, which is a necessary ingredient for making connections and establishing healthy boundaries.

The Fun® Program, EMDR, Brainspotting, and Yoga Nidra all attempt to unveil and access the inner workings and regulating centers of the brain in the psychotherapy session. The evidence-based and not-so-evidence-based practices currently being used in therapeutic settings have radically transformed mental healthcare since I was taught the psychotherapy basics in graduate school. For years now van der Kolk's (2014) best-selling book, *The Body Keeps the Score*, has been *the seminal work* to teach how trauma impacts us and becomes stored in the body. Expanding on this, the founder of addiction Recovery 2.0, Tommy Rosen, claims on YouTube[1] that when we practice yoga, we are literally "squeezing the issues out of our tissues." With so much recognition that trauma, stress, illness, substance misuse, and life events affect the way we think, look, feel, and behave, why are we not spending more time and emphasis in our schools and universities offering courses about anatomy and physiology, especially how the brain works, to everyone? I am still wondering this.

According to brain psychotherapist Bonnie Badenoch (2008), many of our memories (good ones and the ones we don't want to remember) take up residence in our mindbody. She states that we are so conditioned to perceive things only from our left brain (the upstairs brain), that our conscious awareness (the downstairs brain) remains closed until one or several of the five senses (smell, taste, sight, sound, touch) or basic needs (food, clothing, shelter) gets highjacked or "triggered." This is when the subcortical limbic brain (the downstairs brain) lights up and says "Whoa! Where did that come from?" And the upstairs brain says, "Why am I still upset about things that have happened in the past?"

Being fully present in the psychotherapy session, together with the relationship between the client and therapist, will determine the course of the therapy process. At the heart of this is what Grand (2013) refers to as the uncertainty principle: the regulated attuned therapist remains curious about all that is happening, including all details willing to be shared, and intense emotions and sensations that may be experienced (felt sense) and released—all by a process that happens neurologically, organically, somatically, and cortically.

---

1   www.youtube.com/channel/UC-q1peS3J3C9o-uZNXUZ7bw

Gendlin (1982), who coined the term "felt sense," describes this as a physical experience, not a mental one. Merzenich (2013), who refers to himself as "the father of cortical plasticity," explains "cortical" as referring to the cerebral cortex, the thin sheet of brain cells that covers the hemispheres of our forebrains, to which we attribute many of our human powers of perception, cognition, memory, and the control of our actions—where scientists generally locate the "person" at the helm of the ship (2013, p.21).

Flipping our lid

Dysregulation, or "losing it" (losing our mind)—when we are unable to manage and calm our emotions or control our behavior—is now believed to happen due to a culmination of a wide variety of interrelated processes, including the synthesis of internal and external events, emotions, memories, and experiences. Siegel and Payne Bryson (2015) say that when you "flip your lid," it means that your feelings and emotions get so intense that you lose control of your ability to think and act clearly. You may start yelling, kicking, screaming, pushing, throwing things, fidgeting, trying to run away from a situation or avoid it (driving off fast in the car), reach for a joint, go to the bar or casino or mall, feel numb, unable to move, or find it hard to speak. Sound familiar?

This is when the cerebral cortex gets pressured with thoughts like: "Should I stay, or should I go?" Or the brainbody may say and do, "I will think about this later," and then slam the door! When overwhelmed with emotion and experiencing an event as a potential threat (real or imagined), the amygdala takes charge, overriding "rational" thought (the cortical brain), which at this point is not accessible until the regulating centers of the subcortical limbic regions (the downstairs brain) are accessed from the memory filing cabinet of the hippocampus and taken upstairs for consideration from the cortical brain (the upstairs brain). Once calmly regulated, the brain can consider options about how to act and respond, and then the whole brainbody can take a deep breath and calm down.

Let's "think" about or understand this another way. Like the director of a movie, the prefrontal cortex is the complex planner, the deep thinker, and the decision-maker. Packed tightly in the gray matter at the top of the skull, behind the forehead, the prefrontal cortex is the director of your movie called "life." The plot is created from the stimulus obtained in the environment and taken in by one or several of the five senses. When taken in by what is seen by the retina, the information moves via the super pathway (ventromedial prefrontal cortex, agranular cortex to the superior colliculus, taught in Brainspotting trainings) along with input from the other sensory pathways (smell, sound, touch, taste). The superior colliculus is where the storyline or the "plot" gets developed (along with parts of the allocortex, hippocampus, and insula), and characters are created or retrieved (whatever you are reacting to, real or imagined). And depending on which neural networks are being accessed and utilized, the superior colliculus is where, as Del Monte (2023) describes, the structures or "my experience" get created, and the amygdala fires off...or not (fight, flight, freeze, or faint).

Just like sequels to major motion pictures, the original "story" may be over but the script is continuously being revised while the cast and crew members change (the scene changes but the people, places, and situations somehow "seem to be" or may remain the same). This is why, according to Siegel (2002), in the early stages of life, during the establishment of the basic brain circuits that are involved in emotional and behavioral regulation, interactions between the child and social environment are cru-cial for proper development and subsequent functioning. Therefore, during "similar" stressful traumatic situations, the regulating memory recorder of the hippocampus and the amygdala (the alarm center) and other subcortical brain centers may override the executive function of the prefrontal cortex, which has no direct contact with the emotional regulators. In other words, all hell can break loose when the central nervous system cannot calm down, engage the ventral brake, and self-regulate. So, the amygdala keeps sending stress signals (because the hippocampus is saying "this feels familiar, and not safe"), firing off the reactive sympathetic nervous system (fight, flight, freeze, or faint) responses, and we forget how to calm ourselves down (how to chill), because the brain thinks we are in dangerous real time.

Let's look at how Siegel (2023) explains this and why sometimes we may "flip our lid." To easily understand the brain, here's how we can teach young people (and everyone!), using the downstairs and upstairs brain.

> Make a fist with your hand. This is what we call the hand model of the brain. Remem-ber how you have a left side and a right side of your brain? Well, you also have an upstairs and a downstairs part of your brain. The upstairs brain is where you make "good" decisions and do the "right" thing, even when you are feeling really upset. Now lift your fingers a little bit. See where your thumb is? That's the part of your downstairs brain and it's where your really big feelings come from. It lets you care about other people and feel love. It also lets you feel upset, like when you are mad or frustrated. (Siegel and Payne Bryson 2015, pp.55–56)

When looking over this chapter, Amy Weintraub (yoga therapist, author, and founder of LifeForce Yoga®) noted that the upstairs/downstairs illustration is actually a grounding mudra. Mudras, known as yoga of the hands, are gestures used by yoga practitioners (you do not need to be a yoga teacher to use them) (Arora 2015, 2019). Mudras are used to focus and direct energy that can empower clients to use them anywhere, anytime to self-regulate (Weintraub 2012, pp.3, 116). Weintraub explains it like this:

> When we close our fingers over our thumbs, and place the knuckles face down on our thighs, we create what in yoga is called "Adi Mudra," which is like a baby's fist and means "first." Remarkably, for over 1000 years, it has been known in yogic science to evoke a state of "brainbody" calm. (Personal communication, October 18, 2023)

(We will dive into another brainbody yoga practice that regulates the nervous system called Yoga Nidra in Chapter 5.)

And remember, there's nothing wrong with feeling and being upset. That's a normal human experience—especially when your upstairs brain can help you calm down. For example, close your fingers again. See how the upstairs, thinking part of your brain is touching your thumb so it can help your downstairs brain express your feelings calmly. Sometimes, when we get really upset, we can "flip our lid." Raise your fingers up and see how your upstairs brain is no longer touching your downstairs brain. That means it can't help it stay calm.

So, the next time you feel yourself starting to "flip your lid," make a brain model with your hand (remember—it's a brain model, not an angry fist). Put your fingers straight up, then slowly lower them so that they're hugging your thumb. This will be a reminder to check in with your upstairs brain to assess the situation and help you calm those big feelings in the downstairs brain.

I use this hand model often in my practice to show clients how using brain therapies helps us access the downstairs brain in a way that talk therapy technically cannot. While it is important to heal from the neck up, we need to get the whole body involved, so I also talk about how the brainstem is the gateway, the Grand Central Station (like a big train station or huge interstate, with many trains and vehicles coming and going) of regulation, which sends messages to the spinal cord and the rest of the body about how to respond (fight, flight, freeze, or faint).

Siegel (Siegel and Payne Bryson 2015) also suggests we "name it to tame it" (or "frame it to tame it") and "feel it to heal it." We can learn to "name it to tame it" by understanding what happens and developing ways to help the "upstairs brain" get back in control, but we also need to "feel it to heal it." (See Appendix A for a Feelings Wheel that can expand access and vocabulary related to feelings.) Some people have had a tough time growing up (in the family or elsewhere) or have had really stressful experiences in their lives (sometimes called "trauma"). This means that their alarm system can get "stuck" in the "on" position and they can "flip their lid" more quickly. It's not their "fault"—their experiences have made them more alert and on the lookout for danger. For these people, it is often helpful if they practice "naming it and taming it" with a trusted person. This is called co-regulation, attunement, and empathy.

Therapies that focus only on impulsive behaviors, intense emotions, or thoughts may fail to access the deeper processing of the downstairs brain that may need to be accessed for healing. When we have been ignored, cut off, or told "that is not how it happened," to "forget about it," or "stop being so negative," holding the secure space (the therapy session) to focus on and acknowledge the impact of something horrific, shaming, unexpected, dangerous, or life threatening provides the healing mechanism that can occur with an attuned therapist. Here is where The FUN® Program and the other brainbody therapies can be integrated into the psychotherapy session to discover what caused the alarm to go off and keep going off because it "feels" familiar. Siegel (2018) states that mind training, incorporating focused attention, open awareness, and kind intention are the ingredients for creating health, well-being, and happiness in our lives. He created the acronym FACES—Flexibility, Adaptability, Coherence, Energy, and Stability—to summarize how this process works.

The brainbody really does keep the score as well as retaining a ledger, and our whole body will practice what we strengthen (slouching, frowning, yelling, avoiding, crying, dissociating, etc.). Accessing, exploring, and downloading information from the subcortical brain regulators requires more than mental effort and talking alone. It takes willingness (and informed consent) to go down into "the basement" of the brain (using the brainbody therapies) to discover what is stored there, then bring it back "upstairs" so that the cortical brain, now more regulated, can take in information for consideration and gain perspective (how to respond, what to do, etc.). The resourcing and self-regulating practices that occur in The FUN® Program, EMDR, Brainspotting, and Yoga Nidra sessions, over time and with continued practice, can help clients override the pull of the deep blocking (negative, reactive) beliefs and habitual patterns that may be keeping them stuck. Their willingness to be interested in and try these brain therapies and self-care exercises may offer new ways of thinking and behaving, which awakens the brain's own healing capacities to keep us falling and remaining awake (this is our job).

Corrigan and Grand (2013) hypothesize that the brain's orientation to highly emotional, complex emotions, memories, and information involves accessing the orienting response in the subcortical brain. These multiple interconnected systems form an integrated complex network that *cannot be accessed by the prefrontal cortex in traditional talk therapies*. This is where the magic of accessing the windows of the world within the brain begins by studying the movement of the eyes, facial gestures, and body movements/twitching (as is done in Brainspotting and EMDR), but there is more. Sheldon and Sheldon (2022) make the claim that there is a conscious and unconscious emotional brain system, and the hallmark of understanding how these function simultaneously is "like magic." In other words, in as quick as 20 minutes (or less) these systems can enable us to "release the 'rabbits' hidden inside the nonconscious brain systems" (Sheldon and Sheldon 2022, p.27), bringing them to our analytical prefrontal cortex, our thinking and reacting brain. How, you may ask, is this done? Either by establishing the relevant eye position, as is done in Brainspotting, during bilateral stimulation, as in EMDR, or by accessing the deeper brainwave states, as during Yoga Nidra.

What does all this mean?

What this means is that brain regions can regrow due to shifts that occur when these revolutionary therapies facilitate the brain's organic way of accessing and regulating its neural networks. Developments in neuroscience and memory reconsolidation are pointing to relief from presenting symptoms (anxiety, depression, dissociation, stress, etc.), by stimulating and reprocessing memories stored in the hippocampus (Corrigan and Christie-Sands 2020). By studying and understanding the brain basics, and with the practice of brainbody therapies, we know that the brain can change, opening up new hope and relief for much of the distress clients come to us for what was perceived to be "untreatable" (F. Shapiro 2012).

Healing takes place when the new information gained in the therapy session is accessed, processed, and shifted into insights, providing new ways of responding to life. The "work" of psychotherapy and research is creating a shared view of what we now know and are learning about the parts of the brain and how they work as a whole system. This shared view is conceptualizing how the whole body responds to attachment disruption, relational shocks, chronic neglect, and other trauma that can occur during critical periods of brain development and maturation. This is what Maté (2022) refers to as "interpersonal neurobiology" and the reality of our "interconnected nature," concepts coined by Siegel. This goes back to the importance of understanding relationship attachment and disruption and our interconnectedness to each other: "That our individual minds and bodies are intimately connected is fairly simple to grasp...our bodies influence our brains and minds and, necessarily, the brains, minds, and bodies of others" (Maté 2022, pp.54–56).

Neuroscience and our brains continue to evolve as we explore and try new ways to feel happy, secure, and calm, to dream, create, connect with others, and enjoy the delights of life as it is. We now know that the neuroplasticity of the brain has helped us understand that the size and various sections of the brain can be altered and strengthened, depending on the frequency and types of activity the brain is engaged with in the mental and physical environment. The focus on ADLs in healthcare is why we say, "What we practice, we strengthen" and "Use it or lose it," which also applies to all forms of self-care, activity, relationships, and exercise.

We now know we need to do more than just "name it to tame it." Words are important but not enough to access what is going at the subcortical level. According to Lind-Kyle (2010), brain centers change in structure and function by the repetition of mental imagery, emotions, body posture and exercise, and other healthy stress responses such as engaging in novel experiences, learning a new behavior or hobby, or taking a trip. The beauty and adaptability of the innate capacity of the brain to change and adjust to external conditions opens up the possibility for considering different ways of living—for "falling awake." This freedom and power of being in charge of our beliefs and actions invites us to consider new possibilities at every moment (also known as self-reflection, insight, and cognitive reappraisal). As we continue to ponder the biology and origin of beliefs, we can work and rest on hope, knowing that an "old dog" can be taught new tricks at any age—if we want to.

The healing of trauma is a natural process that can be accessed through an inner awareness of the body. (Levine 1997, p.34)

Unfortunately, just because you, your clients (or I) have been to therapy before or "for years" does not mean you, or your clients (or I) are "cured." Trauma, stress, and intense life situations can shove the mind and brain into overdrive at a moment's notice, which is sometimes referred to as "trigger stacking." When self-care or a "time out" is not implemented (you stop exercising, practicing mindfulness practices, going to 12-step meetings, seeing the trauma-informed therapist), the brain can become overwhelmed and link stressful events from the past and present together into one big drama circus. This is when the amygdala alarm center goes off again and the sympathetic nervous system has been informed that you are now in danger as it processes everything together all at once: the screeching of wheels on the pavement, the spray of shattered glass as one car slams into another, the smell of smoke, getting fired again, the teeth of the dog barking, sirens flashing in the dark, a song playing in the supermarket, etc. In other words, the past *feels* present again. A leader in the Kundalini Yoga tradition, Rosen (2014) claims the mindbody release that occurs in a contemplative yet physical practice like yoga gets to the physical and emotional triggers: "issues in the tissues" that can be easily integrated into any 12-step recovery program. This helps us in understanding the importance of what Siegel (2023) refers to as our "embodied brain:" that all these neurons in the brain that grow in complex ways link to the spinal cord, connecting and sending messages to all the major organs and throughout the body.

This may be why in post-traumatic-stress-disorder (PTSD) and other acute mood states it is suggested that what may be occurring is an "existential distress." While not an official DSM diagnosis (APA 2013), people impacted by developmentally adverse events describe themselves as "being stuck" in endless rumination or living in a mental prison, *as if they are still there.* According to Pollan (2018), this could be the result of an overactive default mode network (DMN), or when the chatter and recall of the brain (referred to as the Committee), takes over (Shafer and Greenfield 2000) (more on the Committee ahead!). This activation in the prefrontal cortex is where rumination takes over.

We need to keep the brain processing and evolving. But how? Remember that the brain is resilient! Therapy can become our brain training, and like with a personal trainer, we need to keep working out between sessions (and try different routines). Therapy, I tell my clients, is like a gym: once you have been introduced to the equipment and have been provided with a "work out" or self-care routine, the key, as they say, is to "Just do it!"

Sheldon and Sheldon (2022) suggest (the key word here is "suggest") you ask your clients to do four things right after each session (although even just one will spark the energy of change):

1. Think about and even write down what sensations they felt during the session, such as, "I felt calmer in my chest," "I was able to let go of my baggage and relax my shoulders." Ask what physical movements they will do to access this sensation between sessions if they get triggered—maybe lean back against

a tree, go for a walk, swim, ride a bike, float in a pool, etc. Or if something visual happened, how can they make the invisible visible? For example, if they say, "I feel proud and courageous, like a lion," have them find a picture of a lion and place it somewhere to remind them that they have these qualities.

2. Every morning before they get out of bed, or every time they go to the bathroom, ask them to think about the motivating image they accessed in the therapy session, or just practice calm breathing, or do a gratitude "check in."

3. During physical exercise, ask them to continue to be mindful of the sensations they feel in their body (stronger, confident, happy). You and/or your client can play bilateral music (with headphones on), or music they love as a distracting technique for the busy mind (please stay off the phone though—talking is not part of this).

4. Before sleep, ask them to take an inventory of the day. And to ask their brain to give them a dream to provide insight or answers while they are sleeping.

The brain therapies of The FUN® Program, EMDR, Brainspotting, and Yoga Nidra can offer a mental reboot, a "shaking of the snow globe," to try something different. In addition to "just talking about it" with traditional cognitive-behavioral therapies, the journey taken here will help you explore what nurtures your brain forest—and what keeps you falling awake. Prolonged denial, avoidance, or numbing-out behaviors create unnecessary suffering. Therapists, healthcare providers, and clients sometimes find that EMDR, Brainspotting, and Yoga Nidra can offer more flexible, adaptable methods to get to "the spot" and "finally" experience relief quicker than talk therapy. The unique benefit from each modality fosters the austerity of sound ethical clinical practice: starting where the client is, obtaining informed consent, and trusting that *they* know what is best for *them* (which may require you to refer them to someone who has specified training that you do not have or that goes beyond your scope of practice).

This concludes our guided tour of the brain forest. I hope that this chapter has illustrated how the brain therapies may be able to intervene and help you and your clients to fall and stay awake, providing the brainbody with new and unique ways to access, process, and release difficult emotions—by working in ways in which the brain naturally functions and regulates.

CHAPTER 1: VOCABULARY AND FOLLOW-UP CONCEPTS

Here are some words and topics about the brain for your further study and reference:

- ACE-Q (Adverse Childhood Experiences Questionnaire)
- Amygdala
- Brainstem
- Dissociation
- FACES (Flexibility, Adaptability, Coherence, Energy, and Stability)
- "Flipping our lid"
- Fight, flight, freeze, or faint response
- Hippocampus
- Hypothalamus
- Insula
- Interoception
- Mudra
- Neural networks
- Neuroplasticity
- Parasympathetic/sympathetic
- PVT (Polyvagal Theory)
- Prefrontal cortex
- Regulators of the brain: anterior cingulate, corpus collosum, orbital prefrontal cortex, dorsal lateral prefrontal cortex, ventromedial prefrontal cortex
- Superior colliculus
- Thalamus
- Upstairs/downstairs brain

CHAPTER 2

Welcome to The FUN® Program—Are You Ready to Be a FUN® Therapist?

Over the years, Western mainstream medical treatment and psychotherapy have made valuable and much-needed contributions to our healthcare system, particularly in emergency situations. Having a diagnosis can be the important first step of the healing journey to calm the urgency of the moment. However, meeting with a physician for 10 minutes and getting prescribed medications can sometimes create unnecessary dependency, or only ease the brainbody by getting a temporary "fix." Usually, using medication alone does not substantially alter the "dis-ease" or get to the root of symptom removal to determine what *action* needs to happen *next*. In contrast, The FUN® Program is a cognitive-behavioral approach for healing, created when I co-authored *Asthma Free in 21 Days* (Shafer and Greenfield 2000) and trademarked the program. The FUN® approach to healing introduces curiosity to the cortical left brain: a kind of "wake-up call," not only about what our physical symptoms are trying to tell us, but also about the complexities of our life journey to date, and sometimes the intense emotions and stories attached to these—which is the essence of *Falling Awake*.

Physical ailments and emotional imbalance have been challenging medical science for hundreds of years. However, conventional medicine has yet to look at these "presenting problems" as anything more than a potentially dangerous and discomforting set of temporary symptoms. Modern medicine, such as a 10-minute visit with a primary care practitioner, does not usually inquire, explore, and address the whole person or utilize a brainbody perspective for the office visit. While some healthcare providers are now including the role of environmental, biological, and psychological stressors in triggering and exacerbating symptoms, the brainbody remains barely included as a focus for intervention, symptom relief, and healing.

The FUN® Program is a healing system based on a self-directed, cognitive-behavioral, brainbody approach I created after being hit by a drunk driver while running, training for my first New York City marathon in 1994. At the trauma center where I was transported to, I was told by the medical team that I would never walk again due to the injuries I had sustained (my leg was broken in three places and my clavicle was fractured). In addition, the relationship I was in at the time of the accident was embedded in betrayal and dysfunction, a clinician at my office was being unethical and getting arrested, and now I was possibly not going to be able to finish my PhD. Thinking about all of this while in the trauma center, I started to cry and buzzed the nurse (no trauma or crisis counselor was sent to consult with me). When I told her what was upsetting me, she tapped me firmly on my shoulder and said, kindly, "Shafer, get over it." And then she walked out of my hospital room. That was the trauma intervention I received. So, I thought to myself, "She is right! I can either lie here in the hospital trauma center and keep feeling sorry for myself, engaging in the 'poor me' thoughts, or I could start applying to myself what I teach my clients." This is when I pulled out a pen and paper and wrote down the word "FUN." *Now* it was time for me to really learn what this "accident" was forcing me to look at...this was me falling awake...again—stay tuned.

The FUN® Program emerged from this experience and laid the foundation for *Asthma Free in 21 Days: The Breakthrough Mindbody Healing Program* (Shafer and Greenfield 2000), which discusses my healing journey from asthma. I learned how beliefs become stories we create about things that happen to us. And that by paying attention to what we are thinking and imagining, and by studying the science behind all this is how we fall awake and "make shift" happen. This falling awake process became the guiding principle for my work as a psychotherapist, trauma and addiction professional, and certified yoga therapist.

The approach grew out of my personal and professional experiences with psychiatrist Dr. Gerald Epstein and his teacher Colette Aboulker-Muscat (whom I studied with in Jerusalem, Israel). I first met Dr. Epstein in 1990 through his book *Healing Visualizations* (1989), when I began to use mental imagery as a healing technique to control my asthma triggers (Shafer and Greenfield 2000). After a lifetime of feeling isolated and stuck in my own illness, of being warned away from physical exercise by healthcare providers, Dr. Epstein's belief-based approach and teachings about mental imagery challenged me to gain the confidence to do what I had been told was now unattainable: to run a marathon. A year and a half after my accident, I ran my first New York City marathon without the need of a steroid inhaler or any other medications. I completed it, just as I had always dreamed of, without any of the predicted ill effects. That year, 1994, I was also able to walk on stage to get my diploma for finishing my PhD. I then brought this success into my practice as a social work clinician and educator.

What's FUN® got to do with healing?

The FUN® Program is about lightening up and enjoying the journey while we are still here. We may need to take some things seriously, but it is also okay and permissible to have FUN® and to enjoy the ride. In addition to a refreshing and empowering perspective that is grounded in self-care, The FUN® Program provides fundamental and practical tools for working with uncomfortable feelings and negative beliefs, how to turn our attention toward them, and how to unhook from their influence so that we are free to choose our next actions. You'll find a guide for practicing a few of these tools below and in Appendix B.

In 2014, many years after creating, working with, and sharing The FUN® Program, I was diagnosed with stage 3 breast cancer. I had a double mastectomy, went through chemotherapy and radiation, and am still dealing with inflammation and anaphylactic shock due to food allergies and sensitivities as a result. What The FUN® Program did for me throughout—and kept reminding me—is that my body is an amazing self-healing system. I am now able (and was then) to stay in the present moment when I start to think about and dwell in the past or worry about the future (and stay out of blame, or making up stories about the future). I also pay attention to when the Committee or Monkey Mind may be sneaking in, deepening my inquiry into the beliefs underlying my experience—when it was cancer, or whatever is going on in my life now. The body does keep the score, and the mind does maintain a ledger. When we undertake a brainbody journey to examine the beliefs and stories we are telling ourselves, *shift* happens—we keep "falling awake."

Some not so fun facts about our healthcare system

Complex traumas, illness, and life events know no boundaries—they do not discriminate based on race, religion, sexual orientation, culture, or age. Those who live with complex trauma and illness come from rural areas, small towns, cities, all climates, and a wide range of home environments. None are identical. But they have one thing in common: they leave people scared, alone, hopeless, and not sure where to turn.

More than a billion dollars is spent annually on complicated, life-threatening illnesses within a conventional Western system for healing that is broken (yes, it is). Yet, despite decades of research, the standard medical model can offer us only temporary relief with no healing practices or life management choices to implement. With its focus on preventing and suppressing symptoms using medications and surgery, mainstream medicine has expressed little interest in integrative therapies to support the healing journey along with these medications and necessary surgeries (it is not an either/or approach—it is both/and—hence the words "inclusive" and "integrative"). The light at the end of the tunnel has been obscured by a narrow and limited point of view—one that encourages a submissive role in the healing process. This limited outlook neglects the premise that people can do a great deal more (take responsibility for their health) than medicate themselves only to lessen the severity and frequency of their symptoms or triggers.

It is not surprising that people who have felt powerless within the healthcare system have begun turning to "integrative" and "inclusive" therapies or the very expensive "concierge" medicine (a privately paid "on-call" doctor, where you pay a costly annual fee to have 24/7 exclusive access to a doctor). Unfortunately, our current healthcare system, based on the essentially authoritarian model of expert and patient, has relentlessly perpetuated a victim/compliance mentality. This results in a sense of helplessness, with people wondering whom they can trust and which "authority" can provide the help or answers they need for their own or their family member's healing journey. In this realm, people seeking answers are taught to believe that they should:

- Hand over all important healthcare decisions to those "experts"—some credible and some self-proclaimed.

- Depend only on prescribed medications to prevent, address, and suppress symptoms.

- Refuse to explore and understand the meaningful relationship *to*, or lessons *about*, their illness/diagnosis.

- Consider anything besides "what the experts say" as suspect and/or unreliable.

- Be compliant and accept the treatment plans provided—don't question what they are being told.

Clearly, we need a new approach. I invite you to take in all the information and perspectives presented here and throughout this book with a beginner's mind. Then use what you are drawn to and make it yours. Also ask yourself: Is it the talking therapy or taking the medication that provides the "cure" or heals? Or is it, as I believe and teach, a combination of the techniques presented here (and/or others that you use) that leads to successful outcomes? (There is no right way or wrong way—the choice is yours.)

Here are some basic concepts about healing/therapy/treatment and the therapeutic relationship (between the helper and the one seeking help) that you may find helpful:

- Protect and feel the therapeutic alliance: be attentive, authentic, curious, fun, and helpful—and when in doubt, obtain a consultation (or get another opinion).

- Establish that "something will work"—even if it doesn't make sense now.

- Maintain hope that things do get better or will change—we are doing something that is different.

- Provide new experiences—try something else.

- Arouse curiosity and allow emotions (crying helps many clients, and us, too).

- Enhance competency and confidence in you and your client—keep learning.

Diving into The FUN® Program: take your MEDS!

Most importantly, take care of you—especially the therapists and healing guides reading this! The basic self-care principle of The FUN® Program is "to take your MEDS:" Mental imagery, Exercise, Diet, and Self-care. (This can be anything, including singing along or listening to your favorite music. I personally choose The Rolling Stones, Led

Zeppelin, Madonna, Michael Jackson, and Lady Gaga—and play them really loud!) It is vital to establish daily self-care rituals of some kind. Create priorities by setting aside time for yourself. Strengthening what you practice allows you to teach and guide others authentically.

Rooted in self-care, The FUN® Program teaches you how to wake up and pay attention. You become curious about expanding your awareness regarding the dis-ease you are experiencing. You examine how you are spending your time (watching the news, social media, texting, wandering the internet). You examine how you respond to a crisis or challenging situations. When this process begins, you start to recognize how the roots of core beliefs and emotions create stories that you have made up about your life. Then you can tune in and recognize how the need for freedom and truth influence the mindbody and the reactions taken—you begin to "fall awake."

F = Focus

Focus is the first part of FUN®. Focusing is a process of becoming familiar and paying attention to and intimate with your thoughts, beliefs, attitudes, and actions—and this is the first step of "falling awake." This is done without judging, comparing, criticizing, or becoming attached. You observe and listen to symptoms and mind chatter as valuable indicators—of being awake and curious about what is going on.

Focus reveals the mind–body connection in simple and non-analytic terms through exercises and techniques that bypass the logical, judgmental, distracted mind. It is the first step in the process of paying attention, which is an absolute necessity for genuine healing.

Let's see how this can work. Take a seated position and try this Focus exercise for fun.

FOCUS

1. Take a moment to be still. If you feel comfortable, close your eyes or soften your gaze and gently focus on something in front of you. Quiet the mind.

2. Take a long exhale out through the mouth, a shorter inhale through the nostrils, and increasingly longer exhales out. Do this gently three times just to become aware of your breathing, and land where you are seated. The breath is slow, deep, continuous, quiet, and even.

3. Notice how the Earth is beneath you, holding your body, supporting you.

4. Now in this place of quiet and stillness, give yourself permission to do absolutely nothing for the next couple of minutes except focus on the word "fun." Keep your mind focused on this word only. Pay attention and simply notice what happens during the next few moments of focusing on the word "fun." Try this before going on and reading any further.

WELCOME TO THE FUN® PROGRAM

5. Then, after a few moments, exhale through the mouth slowly and open your eyes.

6. How do you feel now? Did anything shift? What was your experience?

You may have found this exercise challenging, wondering how long you must do this to "do it right" or "make it work." Some of you may have felt the opposite, that it was calming, easy to do; others may have thought, "this is stupid" or "too easy." Or your mind may have been distracted with something else.

Or perhaps the word "fun" was triggering, and you thought that you don't have fun or know how to have fun, or you drifted off into a whole story about the last time you had fun, or the person you are with is not fun, or people, places, and things in your life are not fun, and so on. This kind of distracted thinking is normal when you begin the process of "falling awake." The first step is to stop, pay attention, and notice what you are thinking about: What are you focusing on? If, during the exercise, the thoughts were not fun, what is the belief or story that you are distracted into thinking about? (We'll get in to those later!) If thinking about the word "fun" was not helpful or healthy, reflect and be honest with yourself: What were you thinking about? And what made that so important right now, in this moment?

When you start to pay attention, you are asking yourself and your brain to wake up and reveal all to you—no avoidance, ignoring, or pretending everything is okay. Now you may be saying to yourself, "but that is a 24-hour job." Yes, it is. But know you will go offline, zone out, or fall asleep from paying attention, which again is okay! No judgment! Just keep paying attention, "falling awake," and come back to focusing. When you start to experience symptoms, or find yourself making up stories about the future, just start being curious and pay attention. Or notice that the non-directed, drama-driven mind is just floating around, having triggers that may be taking you into the past or engaging in behaviors that aren't feeling like you are focused on the word "fun." Just notice and come back in to the present and start focusing on FUN®.

U = Undo

Undoing is the second part of FUN®. Undoing goes through the process of undoing thoughts that are not FUN. Doing this is the beginning of the creative process of discovering new ways of thinking, new beliefs about yourself and your life.

The Undo step of the FUN® process stops the default mode network (DMN) and dismantles the Committee. The Committee is a term for the defense mechanisms that keep the DMN in action (the stress response). You will find a full consideration in Appendix B, but for now it is enough to understand that these are the voices within: the Inner Critic, the Procrastinator, etc. Without our even knowing it, it is often the Committee that has been in charge. As you practice, you will learn, realign, and recognize how the stories, drama, DMN, and the Committee have been running your life. In other words, *thinking*, engaging the inner chat room of the Committee, creates the problems. The emotional reaction to this thinking alters beliefs and challenges ways to be kinder, supportive, and patient about your health/self-care journey.

For example, I was diagnosed with asthma at 15 months of age and lived suffering with this chronic "dis-ease" until I discovered and started using mental imagery in 1992. Then in 1994 I was hit by a drunk driver while running and preparing for my first New York City Marathon. During my recovery in the trauma center I created the FUN®. *Then* in 2015 I discovered and was almost killed by stage 3 breast cancer (now in remission). So I have had a lot of time and opportunities to challenge my beliefs and apply The FUN® Program in three very different life-threatening situations. And still do when life hands me new challenges to FOCUS on and see if I am still falling and remaining awake. The asthma is still under control, and I have another emotional therapy dog (Bentley) that I am very allergic to; I am still walking and running (I have run three New York City marathons) and doing yoga (Pilates too); I am now cancer-free and am writing another book (which I never thought I would), during which my mother's health got suddenly worse and she passed away. If I do not continue to apply daily what I have been taught, created, and still learn about beliefs, mental imagery, and lifestyle behaviors, there is no way I could have prevailed and carried on with all this *and* continued my private practice helping individuals, couples, and families.

You've got the power—imagine what you can do! Own it!

The falling awake tools that you will be learning in this book can be used for dealing with:

- Attachments (to people, places, things, beliefs, and being "right")

- Addictions (drugs—legal and illegal, alcohol, codependency, body dysmorphia, gambling, food, shopping)

- Obsessions

- Mental chat room (the Committee, Gremlins, Monkey Mind)

- Mood management

- Cravings

- How to relax

- An emotional meltdown

- Pain management (emotional and physical)

- Anger

- Grief

- Trauma

- Fear/anxiety.

The mere process of Undoing, changing the thought story or belief, into something that feels more fun, puts you in the director's chair—to change the script or "story" that you have and are creating about your life. You can do this since you are in charge 100 percent of the time of what you are thinking and imagining to be true (Epstein 1989; Shafer and Greenfield 2000). This puts a whole new spotlight on how to address symptoms. It is making a priority of recognizing and undoing the core beliefs (cognitions) that are not fun. And since you created them—yes, you—you can change them (but the Inner Critic or Skeptic will need some time to do this). In the exercise you did, focusing on the word "fun," all the distractions, stories, habitual thoughts, and beliefs you created about doing that can be *undone*.

> *If you do not like where you are, move, you are not a tree. (Jim Rohn, 2009, motivational speaker)*[1]

There are four main ways of thinking or imaging behind not having fun. See which one describes what you do (we all have one in our DMN):

- Denial (blaming self or others): Refusing to look at your part or role in the situation creating stress or "dis-ease." The driving emotion in this thinking mode is anger.

- Expectations: Making up stories about the future, maintaining a mental ledger of what we want to see happen when we express something or try something different. The driving emotions in this thinking mode are worry, anxiety, and fear.

- Analyzing: The thinking cortical brain that needs to check out options with "the authorities" or trying to "figure it out" or find answers (mainly on the internet or social media). The driving energy of this way of thinking is codependency.

- Doubt: Regret regarding the past—the "would've, could've, should've, if only" syndrome. The driving emotions of this way of thinking are depression and sadness. Doubt can create illness; we always have the opportunity to do something different.

Appropriately, these four ways of thinking spell the acronym DEAD—as they are stressful thoughts impinging on our immune system (and we all do them when we are not "awake"). These four types of thinking fuel the creation of the false self, known as the Committee (Shafer and Greenfield 2000), Monkey Mind (a concept over 2000 years old), or *Taming Your Gremlin* (Carson 1983)—such as the Inner Critic, the Shamer, the Addict, the Know It All, the Rebellious Teenager, etc. (see

---

1   https://www.brainyquote.com/authors/jim-rohn-quotes

Appendix B). These are defense mechanisms you created to help you cope with what was going on in your life *then*.

This falling awake for me grew initially from my work with Dr. Epstein (1989, 1994), learning about mental imagery, and how powerful our thoughts and beliefs are (he had the original acronym DED, which I then expanded on). Becoming aware of and paying attention to what you are imaging, thinking, and beliefing (yes what beliefs are in charge right now), is the driving force behind the intense emotions and reactive behaviors you may be using to cope. Since you have the power, you can change the images, thoughts, and beliefs you created (and are still creating...beliefing), and learn how to use imagery, thoughts, and adaptive beliefs to heal you and guide your actions *now*. As you start to undo and take charge of what is going on cortically (yes, back to the brain science again), and recognize what behavioral patterns, habits, and ways of thinking and being are not working *now*, it can be a very freeing process to help you fall awake. Just know—change does not happen overnight (you have been doing this for some time). To begin (start somewhere) and make commitment for 21 days (or see what happens in 3-7 days) for changes to start happening and go from there. When we can lose our attachment to expectations and embrace the uncertainty principle (having no investment in the outcome—stay tuned), here you can start living freely and without the need for control. You may notice the capacity to breathe more deeply, experience a sense of calm and less stress, and how to shut down the Committee when they appear. Here is how your ability to stay in the here and now grows. You can remain awake and have fun! There is a saying: The present is a gift, which is why it is called the present.

How do you know when you are not in the present? Because you are not having fun, and the intense feelings, reactions, and behaviors are caught up in one of the four types of thinking. Once this falling awake starts happening, you can address the N of The FUN® Program...*Now what*? What action, movement, or thought can I do that will make my response to what is going on *different*?

N = Now Act!

Now that you are witnessing the presence of a part of you that is falling awake, you may *Now Act* to seize the moment, notice patterns, expand and transform, and bring the program into a live, active experience. Instead of blaming, making up stories about the future, asking the opinion of others, or having regrets about the past, you can now recognize and own that the story you have created is getting old and going nowhere. This is where you say to yourself: Now what action can I do to take charge of what I think and do, gain a new perspective, and begin to fall awake?!

Remember the neuroplasticity of the brain, and that it is possible to keep changing and doing new things no matter what stage of life you are in, what family drama you are still tangled up in, or what real estate you wish you had purchased in another city and moved to. You are not an age, a gender, a race, or a political party—you are a person, and you can do anything you want—remember that the question continues to be: Do you want to live? (I am still here!) Do your beliefs create your experiences, or do your experiences create your beliefs? Keep challenging what you are telling yourself about what you can or cannot do. This is why I call my private practice Limitless Potentials: Here shift happens. I have a huge sign above my office door that I hope my clients read as they exit that says: "Imagine what you can do..."

I love what Cher (at age 77) was quoted as saying when asked: "Don't you think you're too old to sing rock n' roll?" She said: "You'd better check with Mick Jagger" (who had just turned 80 and was still the front man of The Rolling Stones, playing live concerts around the world).

You have now been introduced to the key tools of The FUN® Program—Focus, Undo, Now Act—and the DEAD ways that keep the Committee telling those stories that keep you stuck. This is the healing stance at the core of The FUN® Program: pay attention to what you are thinking about every moment. Know that you have the power to change your thoughts and beliefs (since you created them), and once you do that inner work (stop thinking in a DEAD way, beliefing what the Committee is telling you), you can then choose new ways to act, think, believe, and live. As you work with this, you will naturally be led to consider, "If I am not attached to the beliefs and thoughts that define me, who am I?" Or maybe, "What is my role in this situation? What am I doing?" Or even better, "What is the purpose of my life? Why am I here?" And "How is that going? Who is in charge: me or the Committee?" (Carson 1983; Shafer and Greenfield 2000).

Whatever the issue, concern, trauma, or behavior that leads someone to seek out a mental health or healing arts professional, the first session of contact matters most—it is the first impression and is known as a high impact time (Shafer 2010). If clients can see/feel/sense that you are authentic, attuned, and awake (you are paying attention to them and really care or are interested about why they are there), the tools, format, procedure, protocols, and gadgets absolutely do not matter. What does matter most is what they want from you right now, in this moment. This is why I created this First Session Exercise, which can be used with individuals, families, and groups. If some of the concepts presented here seem too basic or not useful to you, skim over, or even better, take what you find useful here and make it your own.

At the beginning of the therapeutic relationship, it can be helpful to discuss what the client has in mind of what is going to "happen" in therapy. Often something important has changed or taken place just prior to the first session, inspiring them to make the appointment *now*. Helping clients identify their intentions right at the first session can be the essential element in treatment planning and goal setting (also known as case conceptualization).

FIRST SESSION EXERCISE

1. Once you have introduced yourself by stating your name and title (especially if you are agency-based, so that your client knows whether you are a social worker, doctor, nurse, etc.), find out your client's name, age, how they were referred to

you (how they found you or picked you), and what happened for them to call you *now* as opposed to last week, last month, etc. (inquiring about what is the motivation for change or trying something different).

2. Next ask the client if they have ever seen a professional like yourself before. This helps establish dialogue and rapport with you as an educator and collector of information. Sometimes clients don't understand what healthcare professionals in your capacity do, or they have had a bad experience, so this can help demystify and clarify your helping role with them. This works on establishing trust while emphasizing your strict adherence to their privacy and confidentiality.

3. If they have seen professionals like you in the past, ask them if they found it helpful. The focus at this point is for the therapist to pay attention to what the client reports as helpful—and do more of this—and what they report as not helpful. Pay attention, as you want to make sure that you do not repeat what was not helpful for them. Emphasize this with the client. You might even tell the client that this is why you are asking this question, which again is working on establishing the therapeutic relationship.

4. For clients who have never been to a professional, tell them that people who seek out or who are brought to the attention of healthcare professionals are usually experiencing their life being out of balance, or may have had a recent crisis or stressor. There is something bringing them to you that is requiring their attention *now*. This might be something in the mind (intense emotions or thoughts), the body (physical), confusion about a relationship, family, their spiritual life, or a combination of these. Your focus at this point is to help them understand that when the thinking brainbody is out of balance, this is when professional help is sought. You might again ask what is bringing them to you now as opposed to two weeks ago, one month ago, or three months from now, etc.

5. Tell the client that this imbalance is due to a disturbance that is occurring in either the mind (beliefs held creating emotional suffering—leading to "stories"), the body (there is a physical symptom creating distress), and/or spiritually (there are some questions about faith/hope). Continue to tell the client that when a person does not know what to do to bring all this "dis-ease" into balance, they reach out to a professional (therapist, doctor, minister etc.) to determine how to put what seems to be out of order into balance. While you are doing this, hand the client a clipboard or a pad of paper and a pen (this arouses curiosity). At this point, ask them if they have any questions. If they do, answer them, or if they say "no," tell them you would like to ask them a question. Ask them if this is okay with them (establish the "yes" set—which they acknowledge by actually saying "yes" or nodding their head "yes").

   Tell the client your only request at this time is that, until the exercise is finished, you are asking them not to speak or ask questions, that they will have the opportunity to do this when the exercise is finished. (Please make sure that they keep breathing, because they are often paying such close attention to every word that they stop breathing!) Tell them you are going to ask them a question and they are going to respond by writing down one or three answers. Writing down the answer(s) makes the invisible visible. You want to see (literally) what is on their mind. If you are seeing a couple or a family, or conducting a group, give everyone a pad and pen to complete the exercise (this prevents individuals from copying or changing their answer based on what someone else answers). Plain white paper and colored pens is preferred to open the door to client creativity and imagination (keep the experience fun and the client curious!).

6. Ask the client if they are ready (establishing the "yes" set again). When they indicate "yes," tell them you are going to ask them one question and you would like them to write down one or three answers in response. That's right, one or three, not two. Tell them you are interested in the first thought that comes to mind in response to the question. To help them understand, tell them the answer can be in the form of the thought, word, or phrase, and can be as silly or as serious as they like—don't limit the answer.

7. Ask them again if they have any questions before you begin. Tell them that if they are not sure how to answer the question, to look at you and give you a confused look, and you will then ask the question in another way. Then ask, "Are you ready?" The question is, you tell them, "What do you want?" If they try to talk at this point, simply put your finger over your mouth ("shhhhh...") and ask them to please write down their answer(s) and to look at you when they are done. If the client gives you "the confused look" (they still are not talking), simply and gently say: "You came here today because you either want or need something." Then repeat: "What do you want?"

8. Your job as the therapist is to wait patiently. Sit still. Do not distract, talk, or engage the client until they look up and let you know they are finished. When the client, family, or group are all looking at you, ask how many answers they wrote (not what they wrote, not yet). If someone reports "two," ask them to write one more (this may also give you some information about this client, such as if they are having trouble understanding or following directions, refusing to cooperate, challenging rules, directions, etc.) Then ask the client to sign their name and put the date at the top.

Congratulations. You now have the treatment plan, established and created by the client. Have the client read to you what they wrote and tell them this is what you are going to focus on in their work with you.

What makes this exercise quite helpful and useful is that you have just completed several tasks at once. You now know what the client wants (e.g., a treatment contract, your job description); you found out if your client can follow directions (cognitive abilities); a mini mental status was done (is the client oriented to date, time, and place?); and you know if your client can read and write. This exercise also establishes the importance of self-inquiry, modelling the *Focus* component of The FUN® Program. Also, since this was created by the client, it is individualized to the client's wants and needs. Your job in the therapeutic process is to pay attention to what the client wants or needs and to stay there!

Beyond talk therapy

The "history taking" we were taught in graduate school may not be the best way to approach the first session, although it will show up at some point during the therapy process. While it can be helpful in connecting the timeline ("the 10 best and 10 worst memories" can be a way to begin) or doing a genogram to find out who all the characters are in the client's story, the focus on the client's "story" or history has little to do with what is going on *now*, but somehow the past may still be present. The approaches included in this book—The FUN® Program, as well as EMDR, Brainspotting, and Yoga Nidra—can help the therapist (and client) understand how an ample toolbox of brain-based practices are relevant for obtaining optimal mental and behavioral health, while remembering that each person's healing journey is different.

The brainbody therapies work, and all are based on the neuroexperiential model: bypassing the neocortex and going into the limbic brain to "see what happens," regardless of the process or outcome. They all operate on the uncertainty principle (a Brainspotting term), meaning we never know what is going to happen in the therapy session. We just "go with that" (an EMDR phrase) and notice sensations as they come and go without analyzing or commenting (a Yoga Nidra observation). Talking about and getting the story up front can be helpful but is often less important than we have been led to believe. As we will see, these four different practice methods do not require a lot of talking or history taking. They rely instead on the attentive relationship of the practitioner, who is noticing and obtaining information from the client's facial expressions or physical tension, eye positions or gaze while talking, and body posture, sensations, and breathing patterns while sharing the "story."

Early in the therapy relationship (usually in the first session), I engage in psychoeducation with my clients as it is very common that their past is somehow present, or they want to know "how therapy works," what is going to happen, or "How can this help me?" What I may offer for them to consider is that they may be aware of having intense feelings, emotions, or difficult memories, and when these are not talked about, shared, or addressed, they can become the "stories" (they are real but not true *now*) that may be used to protect, avoid, or keep them from trying new ways of thinking and acting—as this has become their "normal." What we are inviting them to think about with The FUN® Program is creating a new "normal," a new way of thinking and beliefing that is not so emotional or reactive. These intense emotions, memories, and the false beliefs created from the past become stories, and, depending on how long ago they happened or how long the client endured something, may have created fundamental ways of looking at life (became their normal), which they believe are real, but are in fact not true *now*. Many clients find those five words very helpful: Real but not true *now*.

In my four decades of experience and training as a psychotherapist, certified addiction professional, trauma expert, and certified yoga therapist, one of the most important questions I ask myself when I am in session with clients is: "What am I doing and why am I doing this?" I am focused on, "How will this help?" this person, family, couple, or group. I also stick to the acronym I learned in Brainspotting: WAIT, for "Why Am I Talking?" I also use WAIT to ask myself: "What Am I Thinking?" Or: "Why Am I Thinking?" Remember, this focus on what we are thinking is the first step of FUN®. (You can also consider WAIST here..."Why Am I Still Talking?" I suggest this to couples and families who don't listen to each other.)

What may be most important to someone when they seek help is that the confidential secure space (the psychotherapy/healing session) is held to tell the story about what happened or is happening to them without fear of being shamed ("Are you sure this really happened to you?"), ridiculed, made fun of ("Oh it wasn't *that bad*"), or told to "get over it"—especially in cases of developmental, generational, and severe trauma. Most individuals, even professionals who are not trained in trauma-informed modalities, don't understand the traumatic responses individuals have—sometimes forever. It is not our job to fix, change, or stop the pain and suffering. We can, however, as trained clinicians, provide the opportunity and means to discover what is keeping someone stuck by bringing it to the surface and finding relief from intense suffering. As leading EMDR expert and author Laura Parnell says: "Enormous energy and tension are employed thinking about and maintaining a psychological past... we believe we are our history. Often after EMDR... The shift is from 'These are my memories' to 'These are memories'" (2007, p.8).

Being clear about our motives, agenda, and intention helps break down and clarify what we are going to do in the therapy session and how. It is not just being "the expert" in a particular format but being attuned to what we are saying or not (WAIT) and why, which questions we are asking, and what techniques we are going to use with the client. If you are a client, you may ask yourself: "If I am stuck or nothing is changing, then what am I doing or beliefing to keep this situation/story going?" You can ask yourself whether you want to change the story, or even consider a new chapter—for a while.

Also, know that Committee members such as the Skeptic and Inner Critic may step in to talk you out of seeing a professional. Maybe they chime in with something like, "This person is a stranger, they don't care about me. I am just another one of their clients." Or, "Why should I tell everything to someone who knows absolutely nothing about me?" Or, "I am too boring, who would care or want to listen to what I have to say?" Notice how the Committee and storytelling takes over when you *Focus* on what you are thinking, *Undoing* the storyline, and are *Now* thinking about doing or trying something different.

Maybe you should talk to or consult with someone?

All of you must be saying this when you read the topic for this section, or "Yeah…I am ready to run to therapy," and you see the long lines outside the therapy office of clients waiting to talk about trauma or things they are upset about. Intense emotions and sad memories can completely overtake us at times, making life feel hopeless and overwhelming. Sigmund Freud, the Austrian neurologist and founder of psychoanalysis, revolutionized how we think about and treat mental health by actually listening to clients and their stories. He presented to us the power of reclining and contemplation by introducing the couch in the therapy office, making it part of the furniture commonly associated with therapy offices to date.

Freud discovered that by just letting clients talk, the unconscious material would bring to conscious awareness the source of the pain, suffering, and choices of behavior. These unprocessed memories and emotions, according to Chödrön (2022), are at the root of our suffering. To move from being DEAD thinkers to falling awake, we need to learn about and access the Committee (defense mechanisms) and the beliefs we've "created," recognize that they are there, and name them. Once we make the invisible visible, we can "see" how much power these thoughts/beliefs/emotions/parts have had over us. Once discovered and made known, we find out what happened and not only why we created them, but also why we gave this way of thinking and "beliefing" the power to keep us "stuck" or from being happy.

However, in life—and what is presented in the therapy office—we reveal how we tend to react in habitual ways that do not permit, or protect us from, this kind of deep exploration or curiosity about what we are thinking about and why. Instead, when we are upset, we engage in the reactive fight, flight, freeze, or faint response with our beliefs, words, or behavior (because this is all we know until this inquiry begins). This is how and why we create a whole storyline to justify and explain why we are thinking the way we are, even with things that happened years ago. This emotional upheaval can also lead to numbing out (with drugs, alcohol, binge eating, compulsive shopping, porn, yelling, throwing things, gambling) and additional efforts to escape the discomfort instead of understanding why we are so upset and acting like "an idiot" (or not a nice person). Engaging in any of these types of reactions repeatedly over time creates habits and builds stories about our lives, which is how these strong negative beliefs are created and run our lives.

Instead of living a life based in shame, blame, fear, guilt, or feeling helpless, try applying the techniques in this book that have been tested over time and based on the science of psychology, neurology, biology, spirituality, and much more. There are many healing modalities to choose from to process life situations constructively. The first step of integrating new life management skills is to acknowledge that all is not okay. Sometimes this self-reflection, awareness, or admitting that all is not well does not occur until something happens to rock our world (a death, diagnosis, accident, arrest, driving under the influence, divorce, suicide, getting fired, etc.), and it may take several things (or time) before we seek help. At this point, our behavior may come to the attention of others, and they may give us the gentle verbal nudge, email, or text to let us know that all is *not* okay with us..."falling awake." You may even wish to consider this Well-Being Scale (Tebb 1995) to "see" how things are going for you:

WELL-BEING SCALE
Basic needs
Below are listed a number of basic needs. For each need listed, think about your life over the past three months. During this period of time, indicate to what extent you think each need has been met. Circle the appropriate number on the scale provided below.

1. Never or almost never   2. Seldom, occasionally   3. Sometimes
4. Often, frequently   5. Almost always

1. Having enough money	1 2 3 4 5
2. Eating a well-balanced diet	1 2 3 4 5
3. Getting enough sleep	1 2 3 4 5
4. Attending to your medical and dental needs	1 2 3 4 5
5. Having time for recreation	1 2 3 4 5
6. Feeling loved	1 2 3 4 5
7. Expressing love	1 2 3 4 5
8. Expressing anger	1 2 3 4 5
9. Expressing laughter and joy	1 2 3 4 5
10. Expressing sadness	1 2 3 4 5
11. Enjoying sexual intimacy	1 2 3 4 5
12. Learning new skills	1 2 3 4 5
13. Feeling worthwhile	1 2 3 4 5
14. Feeling appreciated by others	1 2 3 4 5
15. Feeling good about family	1 2 3 4 5
16. Feeling good about yourself	1 2 3 4 5
17. Feeling secure about the future	1 2 3 4 5
18. Having close friendships	1 2 3 4 5
19. Having a home	1 2 3 4 5
20. Making plans about the future	1 2 3 4 5

21. Having people who think highly of you	1 2 3 4 5
22. Having meaning in your life	1 2 3 4 5

© 1995 Susan Tebb, used with permission from Susan Tebb, Saint Louis University

Unfortunately, the recovery, mental health, and trauma journey with a specialist is often the most avoided, ignored, or dismissed option, considered a stigmatized path to ease human suffering. Many people say, "therapy doesn't work." Trauma, and the words to describe it, such as feeling "triggered," "activated," or "re-traumatized," have become buzz words and phrases used to describe the stresses of everyday life. This is why paying attention to (*Focus*) what we say to ourselves and others about how we are doing and what we are imagining about our life matters, such as, "I am this way because I have ADHD, or PTSD, or anxiety, etc." We do not use the disease or diagnosis to define us, but to help us consider what treatment options we have. Peter Levine (2005), renowned trauma expert and proponent of somatic therapy, stated it this way: "While it is true all traumatic events are stressful, all stressful events are not traumatic" (2005, p.7). Identifying something as traumatic is less important than staying awake and curious about how our intense feelings, emotions, and memories become stories (and beliefs) that now run *our* show—*life*.

Even then, who really wants to go talk to a stranger (especially a professional) about what is going on? And what words do we use to describe it? When there are no words or expression is complicated or avoided, some of the tools and practices in this book can be helpful. Going to therapy does not mean you are mentally ill (we all have "stuff" going on). In fact, like the title of this book suggests, it means you are paying attention and actually wanting to fall awake and do something different. Yay!!!

But you may not know what you want, how to talk about it, or what kind of professional you should see. The first suggestion is to stay present with what is going on with you right now (*Focus*) and learn the lesson of the emotion—consider it a visitor or a gift being handed to you on a silver platter to give you information on what help you need at this time. Trust yourself. Eventually, you will know whether you need or want to seek professional help.

Staying in the present

The ability to be present without reacting, welcoming, and experiencing cravings and urges, teaches clients how to recognize negative beliefs (they do come back) and to act in ways that do not promote immediate gratification. This is called riding the wave of sensation (one yoga tradition teaches the method of breathe, relax, feel, watch, allow). Research suggests that mindfulness tools such as meditation, repetition of a word, phrase, or prayer, or yoga practices along with cognitive behavioral therapy (CBT) can, over time, help control attention and release sensations or cravings to use. The brain-based, trauma-informed practices utilized in The FUN® Program, EMDR,

Brainspotting, and Yoga Nidra help welcome the present moment and develop skills for responding to present events in a calmer way, reducing the engagement of the reactive mind and harmful behaviors (and emotional or behavioral relapse). The practices discussed in this book embrace the understanding that things are always changing and that we can choose to meet, greet, and welcome each moment on life's terms. And how about if we meet and greet others like this all this time? We all have something going on... Let's always practice meeting and treating each other with "nice cream."

A note about the breath. How we breathe really does matter. Research by Nestor (2020) finds that asthma, anxiety, ADHD, psoriasis, hypertension, and sleep disorders, such as sleep apnea, can be reduced or reversed just by changing the way we inhale and exhale. This transformational healing tool naturally occurs every 3.3 seconds (the average time it takes to inhale and exhale). All we need to do is become more mindful about how we breathe.

The nose is the silent warrior that exists in all of us, the gatekeeper of our bodies, the pharmacist to the brain (oxygen), and the weathervane to our emotions. Inhaling gently through the nose invites in cool air, keeping the body calm, making the face look relaxed and beautiful, and even preventing dis-ease. The air that enters the nose gets filtered, unlike mouth breathing, which is like inhaling hot water from a swamp—the choice is yours! The biggest gift of mindful breathing, however, is that it can only take place in the present moment (you cannot be in the cortical brain *thinking* and practice relaxed focus breathing at the same time). Remember, *Focus* on what you are thinking and doing.

Summing things up

Complex thoughts and emotions show up from time to time in our lives. Depending on how much power they have over us, they can lead to negative beliefs and stories we have created that are real but not true *now*. Committee members (defense mechanisms) such as self-judgment, self-criticism (the Inner Critic), panic, anxiety, guilt, shame, or regret were created "at the scene of the crime in the past" to help us cope—but may no longer be needed or are not helpful now. The FUN® Program and other brainbody practices in this book can help us recognize these intense emotions as temporary visitors (we may need to have a meeting with them and invite them to the table), understand what made them show up *now*, and show us how to not unpack their baggage—we do not want them moving in!

Use the steps of The FUN® program:

1. Consider that the thoughts and beliefs you notice when you *Focus* are like suitcases in the baggage claim area. Stick with your own suitcase (mind your own business).

2. Ask: Is there a purpose for this emotion? Is there a need for drama? Is it necessary or appropriate *now*? If you no longer want it, put the suitcase

down (*Undo*)—only examine yours...don't pick up a suitcase that belongs to someone else.

3. Use your FUN® toolbox to *Act Now*: Move, breathe, go to a movie, call a friend, go to a meeting, get a massage, drive to the beach or park, take a short road trip, read, write a story about what's going on, or take some action that feels authentic and correct for you.

Take this thought as we move on through the enchanted brain forest (adapted from the Twelve Steps program from Adult Children of Alcoholics® & Dysfunctional Families[2]): Accept the people we cannot change, the courage to change the one I can, and the wisdom to know that one is me. Now let's go have some FUN® and keep falling awake!

CHAPTER 2: VOCABULARY AND FOLLOW-UP CONCEPTS

Here are some words and topics about The FUN® Program for your further study and reference:

- Change = CCD (Courage, Commitment, Discipline)
- The Committee
- DEAD (Denial, Expectations, Analysis, Doubt)
- False/true self
- Focus
- The FUN® Program
- Gremlin Taming
- Imagination
- Ledger
- MEDS (Mental imagery, Exercise, Diet, and Self-care)
- Monkey Mind
- WAIST (Why Am I Still Talking?)
- WAIT (as in Why Am I Talking? Why Am I Thinking? What Am I Thinking?)

---

2 https://adultchildren.org

CHAPTER 3

EMDR—The Neuroscience Behind Brainbody, Trauma Informed-Focused Care

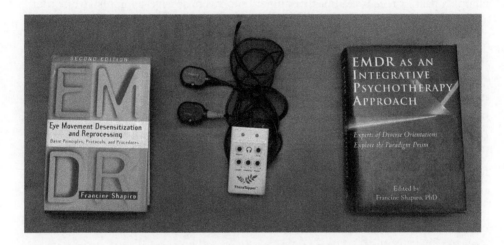

Now that you have entered and started exploring the brain forest and have learned how to be a FUN® cognitive-behavioral therapist, you are about to embark on a new therapy journey or healing path that started with Dr. Francine Shapiro's famous walk in the park (2001, p.7)—learning about the trauma-informed brain therapies, beginning with Eye Movement Desensitization and Reprocessing (EMDR) (Bermann 2012).

It is hoped that as you continue falling awake, learning new ways of providing therapy, or integrating spices into what you already do in your work helping others, this will shift your conceptual framework about complex trauma and other stress-related disorders. What I hope is you will steer around (but not discount) diagnosis and other labels clients come to you with as you *Focus* (yes, the F of The FUN® Program) on treating people who are coming to you with a problem. During this journey it is my hope that you will become excited and curious about the function of the nervous system (yes, the brain) in the treatment of trauma and its role in self-regulation (Kase 2023). First and foremost, please know that some of the exercises provided in this chapter, and throughout this book, are intended to be used in partnership with an EMDR-trained (and in some cases licensed) trauma, mental health, and/or addiction professional. It is also recommended that therapists practice self-care rituals daily, and/or seek help or case consultation from other trained colleagues to clear the entangling energy or countertransference reactions from hearing the stories your clients are telling you (in fact, as I write this I am on a personal retreat).

EMDR, based on Shapiro's eight-phase protocol and adaptive information processing (AIP) model,[1] is an evidence-based approach for the treatment of trauma and other disorders and issues. The theoretical basis of EMDR is the AIP model, which maintains that the primary source of psychopathology is dysfunctionally stored memories of adverse life experiences, stressors in the present, or anticipations about the future that have not been accessed and sufficiently processed by the brain (Keenan et al. 2018). The advances of SPECT scans, fMRI, and our greater understanding of how the brain functions help us understand that clients suffering from severe complex past or recent traumas, or anxiety such as obsessive-compulsive disorder, are not permanently damaged, and that psychological, neurological, and biological changes do take place during and after the EMDR therapy session. Remember—the brain comes with them to the couch!

Unlike cognitive behavioral therapy (CBT) with a trauma focus, EMDR does not require detailed descriptions of what happened, direct challenging of beliefs, extended exposure therapy, or homework (except self-soothing resource techniques called "resourcing" that can be done between sessions when or if a client needs and chooses to). This reduction in history taking, and not talking extensively about what happened, and the practice itself, may at first seem "weird" to a clinician trained in traditional talk therapies such as CBT.

However, the preparation phase of EMDR does include some history taking while clients talk about developmental and recent events that may be helpful to process with EMDR. This phase is done to determine what is referred to as the client's window of tolerance—their ability to tolerate emotions that may be accessed during the EMDR session. According to Leeds (2022), Resource Development and Installation (RDI), which has become a standard part of EMDR basic training, is the psychoeducational part of this phase, which is designed to teach clients how to self-soothe and self-regulate during and after an EMDR session, if needed. Then, once informed consent is obtained and selecting a memory is identified to process, bilateral stimulation (BLS) is selected, often in the form of eye movements, tapping, bilateral sound, or a light bar. And, yes, it is okay if your client moves their head back and forth during the horizontal eye movements with your hand guiding them (please don't point your fingers at them; use an upright hand, about 6–12 inches from the face, determined together along with the seating arrangement—this is all discussed in the basic EMDR training). To activate and put pressure on the neural network for processing, clients may be asked for intensity of emotions while describing the memory in session

---

1   www.emdria.org/wp-content/uploads/2021/08/8-Phases.border.pdf

(therapists watching for activation of the client), noting descriptions of images, sounds, or sensations in the body to be activated for the bilateral brain processing.

Since its acclaim as an evidence-based, trauma-informed clinical practice, licensed therapists undertake intense training and obtain the consultation required to use EMDR in their practice. Because EMDR is not considered a stand-alone therapy, it can easily be integrated into any therapy modality prior to learning and getting trained in EMDR. Remember, EMDR is not a diagnosis-based therapy; it is a therapy based on memory retrieval (accessing), activating the working memory (recalling the most intense/worst part of this), reprocessing towards adaptive resolution (BLS), and landing in the new perspective offered by the regulated central nervous system.

A snapshot of an EMDR session

Let's take a trip back to the brain forest to understand how this works.

> Imagine a forest of trees with trails running throughout it. The trees represent memories and the trails through the forest represent memory networks. Trails traveled frequently are well defined and quick to access, while trails seldom traveled are less defined and more challenging to identify and access. Building new trails is possible but requires tools and effort. This process takes time and patience because a new path has to be carved out, tended to, and frequently traveled, before transforming into a well-defined trail. (Kase 2023, p.61)

Kase is saying is that transformation takes time, practice, and trusting the process that change can and is always occurring. Every time a client comes to see us, they are bringing in new memories, new data, along with the thinking mind to challenge these new neural pathways (new ways of thinking and beliefing). Stickgold (2002) also used the forest analogy to explain the action that occurs in an EMDR session.

Here is a summary of what the first EMDR session can look like.

The client comes to your office with a presenting problem or was referred to you (you may ask why they chose EMDR, what made them seek this out at this time). This is briefly discussed, which includes how EMDR can be helpful and what can happen during an EMDR session:

- Clients are told they will choose an event or memory to work on and discuss how upset they are about it now (using a Subjective Units of Disturbance Scale (SUDS)).

- Eye movements, known as bilateral stimulation, will be used in the form of (and demonstrate this) the eyes following the hand in front of the face (sometimes fast, sometimes slow, sometimes changing directions) (Andrade, Kavanagh, and Baddeley 1997).

- Or tapping on the body will be used (which you demonstrate) or tappers held in their hand, or a light bar (show them if you have the tappers or light bar).

Clients are also told that sometimes during processing, intense memories and feelings may come up (for "no apparent reason"), and if they choose they can stop the session by just raising their hand (the STOP signal), letting the therapist know they wish to pause and process.

Unlike traditional talk therapy, instead of engaging in dialogue it is suggested that if the urge to do this arises during BLS, that the client continues to let the EMDR do what the research has found helpful—accessing and bringing up the intense feelings and memories, and then letting them go. I tell clients that it is like driving a car through a dark tunnel: What happens if you take your foot off the accelerator? You stop and are stuck in the middle of a dark tunnel! Therefore, I suggest they keep their foot on the accelerator until they get through to the end, as there is light at the end of the tunnel—meaning that the intense feelings will be released and they will feel calmer at the end. I also remind them that there is no right or wrong way to experience an EMDR session—whatever happens, or not, is what is meant for them at this time. I also remind them that EMDR is not a single session therapy (although a lot can happen in just one session), or a replacement for taking medications or other forms of medical care they are currently involved in. This is why EMDR is considered an integrative, trauma- and neuro-informed psychotherapy (Lee 2020).

However, we want the client to feel that they do have control or some say in what happens in session, so explaining the use of the STOP signal is very important. If this is understood, all questions are answered, and they agree to EMDR, then the client provides signed informed consent to engage in the EMDR session. Once this is completed, a "target" or memory/stressful event to process in the EMDR session is chosen, knowing that several sessions may take place to determine this if they are not sure—there is no rush to transformation! This can include processing traumatic memories or stressful events of the past or present, or working on anticipations they have about some future event.

As the client settles in and begins to think or talk about the memory/issue, they are introduced to the different options available to experience BLS. Sometimes clients ask me, "Which one works the best or produces the fastest results?" I remind them that the idea is to anchor the brain in the current moment as they recall the stressor of a past event or current issue, known as the process of dual attention stimulation (Shapiro 2010, p.32). I tell them the "best bilateral stimulation or use of eye movements is what they prefer" (the research suggests using the original method of the fingers going back and forth). During a virtual telehealth EMDR session clients might physically cross their arms and tap alternate triceps, watching the therapist on the screen and doing it together (also known as Butterfly Hug or Angel Wings); they can also listen to bilateral music[2] on headphones; or they can have "tappers" for each hand (or put them in their pockets).

The EMDR sessions provide individuals with a nonverbal, somatic, effective way

---

2   Bilateral music is a type of music that you can listen to using headphones, where you can hear the music alternating between the left and right ears, using dual attention focus (listening to the sound while the eyes are engaged with the BLS).

to reprocess the painful memories stored in the amygdala (the trauma/drama-holding center in the mid-brain). Once again, the amygdala is the alarm center igniting the fight, flight, freeze, or faint reaction that seeks to protect us, informing us that we may be in danger. Memories that are not fully processed can create "unique" neural networks that, when triggered, may lead to flashbacks, nightmares, dissociation, and other disruptive emotions and behaviors in efforts to self-regulate. The memory processing that occurs during EMDR helps calm the amygdala by releasing these dysfunctionally stored intense feelings and memories to help shed light for the client to process, finding new perspectives or the source of their reactive responses. Known as DAS, during processing of emotional content, the eye movements seem to have a direct effect on cognitive processes (Shapiro 2002, p.372). This is the process where once the memory/issue chosen to be the focus for the session is determined, the client is asked to think about the worst part of the event (memory), to establish the negative belief they have about themselves associated with this, how intense or activated they feel as they think about this now on a scale of 0–10 (where 0 = no distress and 10 = very distressed, called SUDS), and sometimes, if appropriate, exploring where they feel this in their body. They may also be asked when they think about this disturbing event and what happened, to describe how they would prefer to believe about themselves instead, which is called taking a Validity of Cognition (VoC): "When you think about this event now, how true does this preferred belief feel to you now, on a scale of 1–7 (where 1 = not at all and 7 = feeling totally true)?" The eight-phase, unrestricted EMDR processing, and others (EMD, EMDr), are structured to access and work with the associated memories, intense emotions, beliefs (stories), and sometimes physical sensations (Schwartz and Maiberger 2018; F. Shapiro 2012).

Shapiro found that after desensitization, not only did clients report feeling less disturbed (the SUDS went down), but they also felt more confident and possibly able to embrace the preferred belief they identified to work on during treatment planning. She called this process the AIP model, which is defined as the brain's innate ability (neuroplasticity) to light up different neural processing networks—"falling awake!"—during BLS. This, along with the attunement of the skilled therapist, helps the client recognize that the painful events and negative beliefs about them *are real but not true now*. The event(s) are over, and they are in a different place in their life *now*—somehow, they made it *here, to the present*.

Licensed clinical therapists who have completed the EMDRIA-approved basic training conduct the EMDR session in the eight phases or steps developed by Shapiro. She originally suggested EMDR that typically takes from 6 to 12 sessions to process traumatic events. While the number of sessions required to complete "the work" varies from person to person, she recommended each session last between 60 and 90 minutes. However, much can be accomplished in the standard 50-minute session and may be all the client (or you) can handle or need. And single or two-session EMDR therapy is possible, depending on the need of the client and the appropriate training and skill of the attuned therapist.

Eye movement and the bilateral brain

When Shapiro developed EMDR in 1987, she was grappling with her own disturbing memory. Experimenting on herself, she found relief by flitting her eyes back and forth while thinking of something upsetting, a technique she discovered during her famous "walk in the park." Initially focused on the treatment of PTSD, EMDR was later adapted by Shapiro and others for working with past memories, depression, mood disorders, addictions, anxiety, phobias, current stressors, or intense fears about the future—embracing her AIP model.

In *The New York Times* article "'One Foot in the Present, One Foot in the Past:' Understanding EMDR" (2022), Blum describes how trauma "shoves the mind into overdrive. The brain tries to block out fragments of the disaster" making the reactive and emotional client unable to consciously talk about and understand why intense memories or situations are upsetting them *now*. EMDR (Eye Movement Desensitization and Reprocessing), developed by Dr. Francine Shapiro, pioneered the way of bringing evidence-based, novel, unsupported therapy into mainstream treatment for trauma. In recent years, EMDR has attracted more attention and increased demand for this kind of therapy since the Covid-19 pandemic and thanks to celebrities (Prince Harry, Sandra Bullock, Jameela Jamil, etc.) going public and sharing about the help they receive from EMDR therapy.

Shapiro developed EMD in 1987 and wrote her first paper on what she was discovering about how the processing of stress occurs in the brain between the parasympathetic and sympathetic nervous system. Later calling it EMDR, she said it worked by asking the client to think of a troubling memory or issue, then would hold a pencil in front of the person's eyes, and move it back and forth (bilateral stimulation, BLS) rapidly in a horizontal line (left to right) asking the person to follow the pencil with their gaze as it moved back and forth. She explained that this process helped "balance the hemispheres" as the phobic or trauma response was due to "hemispheric imbalance in the brain." (Frausin and Grinder 2017).

In the late 1980s, neuro-linguistic programming (NLP) had become popular and included the gem of knowledge that eye movements in different directions are associated with different kinds of brain processing. It is speculated that Shapiro, trained in NLP, knew about eye accessing cues before she came out with EMDR (she worked in John Grinder's office in the mid-1980s for about a year before her "discovery" of EMDR). It is also thought that the eye movement process during REM (rapid eye movement) sleep mimics the brain processing that happens during the EMDR session.

During BLS, both hemispheres of the brain become involved (distracting the working memory or cortical brain), alternating the eye movements quickly from one side to the other (or in other directions) so that other memories or insight can be obtained. The thinking cortical brain gets "stuck in the story" and the BLS overrides this protective part that may not "want to go there." According to Parnell (2008), you can also conduct BLS by tapping on your legs or knees like drumming (the client and therapist can do it together) and/or by lifting the feet up and down, like marching in place, tapping each side one at a time. Some people prefer these options, and they can close their eyes to put more *Focus* (like in The FUN® Program) on what they are experiencing, instead of having to look at the therapist.

Again, the theory behind BLS is to bypass the rational left brain (remember the prefrontal cortex from Chapter 1, the part of the brain that tries to figure things out?), access what is stored in the subcortical brain and overworking the amygdala (the alarm center), release the images, thoughts, and memories creating the fight, flight, freeze, or faint response. You may also remember from Chapter 1 that according to Schwartz and Maiberger (2018), the limbic brain structures central to the production and expression of emotions are the thalamus, hypothalamus, amygdala, hippocampus, and the anterior cingulate cortex (ACC). While the field of neuroscience is still evolving, the research in neuroimaging of SPECT and EEG scans points to enhanced left hemisphere function, increased limbic activation, calmer, less reactive, cortical activity, and increased activation of the ACC (the regulating centers of the brain) after an EMDR session.

According to Porges (2017, 2022), creator of the Polyvagal Theory (PVT), known as the science of feeling safe (mentioned in Chapter 1), many mainstream therapeutic strategies (such as talk therapy) separate feelings from concurrent thoughts and behaviors. Porges says that using therapies that are PVT-informed focuses on enabling the client to just notice and experience the feelings without linking these to thoughts and behaviors (Dana 2018). In other words, with this brainbody approach, clients during the EMDR session learn that the feelings are not intentional or under voluntary control but are part of a larger, complex adaptive process, embedded and wired into our nervous system. These findings suggest that the bilateral processing in the EMDR session increases the client's ability to reflect on traumatic, stressful material or fears about the future—referred to as the "intolerance of uncertainty" (Keenan *et al.* 2018). This dual attention (staying present while processing, like watching a movie on a screen) prevents over-stimulation due to the regulation that is occurring simultaneously in the limbic and parasympathetic systems (the past or uncertain future is not present *now*). The balancing function of top-down and bottom-up processing of the brain strengthens relief from the distress associated with disturbing memories. The relaxation response obtained by BLS/DAS suggests that the action of EMDR processing orients the client's attention to be present, as there is no current threat in the moment.

The evolution of EMDR

Over time EMDR has evolved from being referred to as an "unorthodox treatment" to being regarded as the gold standard of "evidence-based" trauma-informed therapy. While some still consider EMDR an "emerging therapy," its esteemed reception worldwide as an integrative trauma-informed practice makes a compelling case for acceptance in the mental health world and has opened the door for other NUST (novel unsupported therapy) supporters to get trained in EMDR and try it. EMDR therapy has become known as a "neurological approach," involving and alerting the brain that, yes, you are upset, and what happened was awful and not okay, but that it is possible to consider new ways of thinking and feeling about what happened *now*. This includes how to turn on the ventral vagal, so that the sympathetic and dorsal systems can calm down and relax, and the client can feel better inside.

EMDR, known initially as an effective form of trauma therapy for PTSD, has now been adapted to address many behavioral health concerns. For example, Robin Shapiro (2020) created parts work, which addresses complex ego states that get stuck in the brain's neural network and are unable to connect with the adaptive, regulated, present-oriented awareness. While CBT ("talk therapy") helps clients cope with symptoms, EMDR brings what is intense to the surface, accesses the working memory for processing, and once activated can provide the resourcing and self-regulation to calm down and gain a new perspective. There is also recent clinical evidence and research to support that EMDR can be highly effective in reducing the compulsion or urge to engage in many destructive behaviors, such as alcohol and drug abuse, self-harm (cutting), domestic violence/anger management, control of obsessive-compulsive thinking, disordered eating, nightmares, complex stress, and more.

The international association for EMDR, known as EMDRIA, is the governing body overseeing what constitutes an EMDR clinician, and maintains strict guidelines on what EMDR is and who can use it in clinical practice. This is because EMDR is more than just waving your fingers in front of someone's eyes, having them tap on their body or hold tappers to "see what happens," then, when they tell you what is happening, you respond by saying, "Great, go with that." It requires someone to be a licensed psychotherapist first; only then can licensed therapists take the formal EMDRIA-approved training and complete the necessary consultation hours after the basic training course (Abel and O'Brien 2015).

Many experts in EMDR have taken Dr. Francine Shapiro's original works (1995, 2002; Shapiro and Forrest 1997), put their unique thumb print on it (while respecting and adhering to her original concepts), and have taken it out into the world to help those who have been profoundly wounded by traumatic or stressful events. Here are a few of them (some I have already noted, and there are many others; and those listed here are not in any special order):

- Grand (2001, 2013), originally an EMDR therapist working with performing artists and athletes, developed what he calls Brainspotting (where the eyes go, energy flows—stay tuned).

- Parnell (2013, 2018) created attachment-focused EMDR, which emphasizes the type of attachment that did or did not happen in a client's childhood or other stages of life. She also adapted EMDR for work with addictions.

- Shapiro (2005, 2016, 2020) ignited what is known as Ego State Therapy (also called parts work), and has introduced us to many EMDR experts and ways of using EMDR in her EMDR Solutions series (Volumes 1 and 2), as well as how to "do" psychotherapy.

- Knipe (2019) and Forgash and Copeley (2008) also contributed to Ego State Therapy (known as parts work with trauma and dissociation).

- Kiessling (2005) introduced his integrative belief-based, resource-development strategies approach to the healing processes in EMDR.

- Marich (2011, 2012, 2023; Marich and Dansinger 2018, 2022) brought her understanding of EMDR for addiction issues and integrated it with 12-step recovery, demystifying dissociation by sharing her personal journey (Hensley 2016).

- Schwartz and Maiberger (2018) combine EMDR with somatic (body-based) psychology.

- Kase (2023) teamed up with Porges (2022), introducing us to Polyvagal-Informed Therapy.

- Leeds (2016, 2022, 2023a, b), psychologist and marriage and family therapist, developed the Resource Development and Installation (RDI) protocol, and contributed to the evolution of EMDR through his publishing and EMDRIA-approved training and consultation at his Sonoma Psychotherapy Training Institute and at workshops internationally.

In recent years EMDR has become "popular," gaining notice in part due to increased demand for trauma treatment during the Covid-19 pandemic lockdown. On-demand virtual sessions became a safe haven for people unable to seek help live, and provided unprecedented access to many new to seeking help. Additionally, well-known people and celebrities, such as Lady Gaga, and Justin Bieber, came forward to share in the media how they found help with EMDR, reducing the stigma of seeking help from a therapist. For example, in a documentary series with CNN reporter Anderson Cooper and television host Oprah Winfrey, both Prince Harry and actress Sandra Bullock shared how they were helped by EMDR—Prince Harry for coming to terms with the death of his mother Princess Diana, and Sandra Bullock after a stalker broke into her home. *The Good Place* actress Jameela Jamil wrote in a 2019 Instagram post: EMDR "saved my life." David Beckham is a former professional soccer player and current model and philanthropist. In his 2020 documentary *David Beckham: Into the Unknown*, he revealed that he had used EMDR to address his anxiety and fear of failure. Beckham said that EMDR helped him "unlock certain emotions" and "move forward" in his life.

Why use EMDR for individuals with trauma?

Most people don't show up to therapy saying "Hey! I want to work on all my traumas: the divorce of my parents, the bullying I endured during grade school, and the death of my pet." They usually start off by saying "I don't know how to start therapy but I'm miserable" or "My drug and alcohol use is out of control" or "I am scared about my upcoming surgery."

During the first clinical interview, the EMDR practitioner will usually discuss the current challenges bringing the person to the appointment, gather the most pertinent information and paperwork, and then might suggest using EMDR as part of the client's therapy journey. It is important to emphasize that there may be more work to be done prior to and beyond the first EMDR session. This can mean EMDR may not be introduced right away, or even at all. It can be helpful to remember and to tell clients that what is disturbing them did not happen "overnight"—it took them some time to think about and make an appointment. This point is raised by Leeds (2022, 2023a, b) who created the Positive Affect Tolerance and Integration (PAT) protocol (Korn and Leeds 2002). He noted that some survivors of early childhood trauma and neglect have difficulty accessing and tolerating moments of appreciation, praise, feeling confident, and the ability to enjoy or receive affection, which can show up in the session. In such situations, alternate EMDR therapy tools may be needed to overcome defenses created from lack of exposure to secure, developmental attachments, which could block the benefits that may be obtained by standard EMDR therapy.

At this first session, the client and therapist may devise coping strategies for the client (known in EMDR resourcing), such as breathing exercises, tapping, movement, or other calming and self-soothing strategies to manage sudden insights, disturbing emotions, or intense dreams that may occur during or between sessions. These calming techniques can be helpful to introduce during the therapy session and reviewed again later to use if something similar happens in the future and they need to calm down. These mindful exercises can be helpful, as the brain may continue processing what happened after the therapy session (like thinking about a movie they have just seen). Shapiro developed the acronym TICES as a guide for clients after an EMDR session: "notice what Thoughts, Images (dreams), Cognitions (negative/preferred thinking, challenging beliefs), Emotions, and Sensations (emotional, physical) occur after the session as you go about your life." (Shapiro 2001, p.429; Hensley 2016, p.132.) These between-session processes can also be used as possible "targets" or "topics" to be discussed at the next EMDR session.

Remember, before the EMDR session, it is important for the client to know that they can stop the session and talk at any point. This reminder (said several times, like in this chapter) is to signal to the therapist that they want to stop the session or talk. This can be for any reason: to provide additional details or history about their current symptoms; to explore what just "came up;" or what they are thinking about during processing, such as a recent emotional outburst, panic attack, or relapse, so they can isolate the triggers that provoked it. A client may also want to ask the therapist questions or to share about other points in their life when they felt like this. One goal of the EMDR session may be to identify how long the situation has been going on or how it feels "familiar," to recognize why things are so disturbing *now*.

When the client understands how EMDR works and what can happen (no surprises), the therapist instructs the client to identify what they want to work on (the memory, event, or issue), known in EMDR as "the target," for the session, and they invite the client to describe the most difficult aspect of this issue. Once shared, the therapist asks, "As you think about what you just told me, what is the worst part?" It could be an image, sound, smell, touch, or taste that allows the intensity of the issue to be revealed. Each person is unique when it comes to feelings or sensations. After the client answers, the therapist can ask for the Subjective Units of Distress Scale, or SUDS: "While thinking about this incident/memory/situation, how intense does this feel for you now on a scale from 0–10...0 meaning no distress or disturbance at all, to 10, very distressed?"

Once the level of distress is determined, the client might be invited to notice where they feel these sensations in their body (it may be one place or more). During some setups for EMDR, the therapist may help the client identify thoughts associated with the issue being addressed, known as the negative cognition (NC) or belief about the event ("I am not good enough," "It's my fault, I should have done something"). Then they may also be asked what they prefer to believe about the event instead ("I did the best I could," "I am okay," 'It's over; I survived"). Both can be reprocessed during the EMDR session with the therapist's assistance using BLS.

Then, having obtained informed consent to use EMDR to "open up" the agreed memory/situation/trauma/dream (past, present, future), and the type of BLS (eye movements, tapping, etc.) is chosen, clients are asked think about the chosen issue tied with the NC, and to notice what happens or what they are experiencing as they engage in BLS (moving their eyes to the left and the right while they watch the therapist move their hand back and forth at eye level, tapping on their body, or hearing faint beeping sounds, with the use of headphones, that alternate between their ears, etc.). Each "set" of BLS typically lasts between 30 and 60 seconds (it is common to do 10–15 passes at a time).

Between each set, the therapist will stop the BLS and invite the client to take a breath and exhale, "Let it go" and to then tell the therapist (if they would like to) what they are noticing or feeling. Whatever the client says, the therapist says, "Go with that" or "Notice that."

Pushing a patient to deliberately revisit the past is not the primary feature of EMDR. During EMDR, the added component of BLS anchors the patient in the current moment as they are engaging with a recent or past trauma (known as dual attention). The phrases "The past is somehow present" or "One foot in the present, and one foot in the past" describe what happens during reprocessing in EMDR. The brain does not have the capacity to completely focus on both the BLS and the traumatic memory. The theory behind EMDR is that memories become less vivid and emotional when a client can't solely focus on them. BLS seems to be compelling enough to distract clients, but not so overwhelming that they totally focus on it, opening up new neural pathways for the brain to consider and gain new meaning about what happened and how they got through it.

More adaptions of EMDR

It has been repeatedly shown that EMDR sessions can knock the neural networks out of flashbacks, looping, and dissociation, to move toward stabilization and access to cognitive processing. The original eight phases have been adapted by leading EMDR experts, authors, and EMDR trainers to accommodate various presenting problems, complex traumas, and emergency situations.

Among this for your further review and EMDR training is what is called the Processing Continuum[3] (EMD-restricted, EMDr-contained, EMDR variations of the original EMDR), created in 2006 by Kiessling.[4] Gomez came out with her very creative and innovative *The Thoughts Kit for Kids* (2008), and My Helpers and Protectors using EMDR age-appropriate phrased card decks to use with children and teens impacted by trauma.[5] Paulsen (2017) wrote and developed her EMDR neurobiological approach for dissociation with early trauma and neglect held in implicit memory. In 2021, Matthijssen and colleagues developed the controversial but popular EMDR 2.0, with others also using integrative approaches (Dominguez 2022; Manfield *et al.* 2017), including the Floatback technique developed by Browning (1999); combining EMDR and schema-focused therapy from Young, Zangwill, and Behary (2002); cognitive interweaves (Shapiro 2001); and Ego State Therapy (Forgash and Copeley 2008; Shapiro 2016). And if all else fails regarding when to use any of these modifications or interventions, please obtain case consultation or use Luber's (2010) EMDR scripted protocols as a guide and to strengthen your knowledge and confidence about how to use EMDR.

Trauma and EMDR

It's not about the power of the substance or the addictive behavior. It's about the power of the pain beneath it. (Hope Payson, LCSW-EMDR, LADC, Trainer, Creator and Director of the film Uprooting Addiction: Healing from the Ground Up, *quoted in Dansinger 2019)*

The Impact of Events Scale (IES) (Weiss 2007) and the Adverse Childhood Experiences Questionnaire (ACE-Q) score (Felitti *et al.* 1998) can tell us how trauma has affected a person's life. The answers to these questions can help us and our clients have a greater understanding about what constitutes trauma and the impact on the brain (memory storage, protective/reactive defenses created) and themselves at the time of the trauma. Bringing to the forefront what exactly happened, and discussing their answers to the questions, can shine a spotlight and provide some insight, such as: how long it occurred, and what, if anything, was done about it (did they try to

---

3 www.emdria.org/course/using-the-emdr-processing-continuum-emd-emdr-emdr
4 https://emdrconsulting.com
5 www.anagomez.org/product/the-thoughts-kit-for-kids; www.anagomez.org/product/my-helpers-and-protectors-therapeutic-cards-that-work-with-the-self-protective-system-of-children-affected-by-trauma

tell someone about it), as well as self-understanding—"No wonder I feel/think/act this way!" Despite the effect of these in validating the impact of trauma, it remains surprising how many mental health professionals do not know they exist or what it means to have a trauma-informed practice (Spence 2021).

Paulsen (2017) says in her book *When There Are No Words* that EMDR can access those parts of the brain that traditional talk therapy cannot access:

> Neocortical learning includes coping strategies, functional capacities, and social skills, and other knowledge and understanding about emotions. Traditional talk therapy most often works on this level. Cognitive behavior therapy attempts to change the affect from top down, by examining beliefs and experimenting with alternative beliefs and conclusions, practicing new behaviors, and not being led by other's emotions. EMDR therapy and somatic therapies tend to work from the bottom up, processing affect, which potentiates subsequent cognitive shifts, either spontaneously or with assistance from strategically timed brief cognitive interventions. (2017, p.74)

It can be challenging to determine the method that "works best" when individuals come for help with PTSD and complicated stress histories (accidents, surgeries, deaths, life-threatening illness, divorce, addiction, domestic violence, discrimination, war, terrorism—see the IES). Evidence-based practices that are indicated and recommended for working with acute stress and complicated traumas include Exposure Therapy, CBT, EMDR, Brainspotting, Yoga Nidra (which you will be reading more about), and when indicated...medication management. Given the client's right to self-determination and to be treated as a unique individual, diverse, creative, somatic interventions such as these should be considered, given the variety and depth of issues brought into to the therapy session.

Psychoeducation may also be needed with a client, such as an explanation of trauma symptoms or other trauma responses such as flashbacks, insomnia, disordered eating, chronic pain, loss of memory, intense feelings and emotions (need for drama), panic attacks, shame, guilt, addictions, anxiety, depression, and dissociation. This is so clients understand that trauma responses are *normal* in such situations and may have been used as a coping tool. The EMDR therapy session can become a secure, reliable space to talk about and learn from all that happened to them without engaging the fight, flight, freeze, or faint response. Understanding that the trauma or incident is over and learning how to release feeling while being present in the EMDR therapy session is when the journey of healing and transformation begins.

Trauma responses occur when the brainbody does not know how to self-regulate and calm down. According to Forbes (2011), and van der Kolk (2014), it is not helpful for people who have experienced trauma or stressful situations of any kind to just simply talk about it, but rather, they need to be involved in some kind of behavior change or movement. When people become physically involved in their treatment, they begin to realize that they have choices and can take control of themselves again. Talk therapy is needed for those who have been traumatized, and is more successful if combined with some type of action, physical exercise, or brain-based therapy. According to Forbes (2011, p.xiii): "Conceptual insight is not required for some change; in some cases, it actually interferes with it. By working in a body-based realm, we can bypass this emotional interference. Much of the healing occurs when the individual begins to develop a relationship with one's body, bringing the brainbody together."

Van der Kolk makes reference to Charles Darwin and his book *The Expression of the Emotions in Man and Animals* (1872), stating that like animals, if we humans stay stuck in survival mode our energy remains locked in fight or flight, focusing on fighting off unseen enemies, which leaves no room for allowing in nurture, care, and love (2014, p.76). A body that is moving and working/functioning properly is a body that is effective—running efficiently. The brain is the organ to get the muscles to move (lengthen and relax) and they involve the vagus nerve, otherwise emotions get stuck in the amygdala (brain basics again). When these memories or feelings are not in conscious awareness, this is where numbing out can happen by using substances or other behaviors (shopping, gambling, overeating) to calm sensations in the brainbody.

Here are some suggestions on how to process the trauma response:

- Regulate the physiological arousal: Utilize calming techniques such as mental imagery to slow down the heart rate, relaxing the breath, and cuing to notice sensations and posture in the physical body (arms, hands, legs, shoulders, back, and feet).

- Access the subcortical brain: Acute stress disorder, which is a precursor to PTSD, is a string of symptoms/incidents that become linked together. EMDR is a technique that can access and bring to conscious awareness intense memories stored in the brainbody.

- Utilize the body, as in Yoga Nidra (or exercise that involves movement), to learn how to occupy the body and the mind. According to van der Kolk (2014, p.273): "If you are not aware of what your body needs you cannot take care of it."

In *The Body Keeps the Score*, van der Kolk recommends EMDR as one of the most effective ways to combat PTSD symptoms, adding: "It's not really an innovative treatment anymore. It's something that's very well-established" (quoted in Blum 2022). Van der Kolk and neuroscientist Damasio (1999), Porges (Porges *et al.* 1994) and others mentioned earlier (back to the brain forest, Chapter 1), embrace how changes in emotional states accompany shifts in physical sensations. However, most forms of traditional talk therapy continue to focus on the meaning of emotional states (cortical processing) and ignore expressions or changes in the physical body. Since we are subcortical creatures, especially traumatized people who are at the mercy of their sensations, physical reactions, and emotions, self-regulation begins at the brainstem—a part of the brain that is essentially hidden from conscious awareness and cannot be calmed or soothed by reason (Blum 2022).

In England, the National Institute for Health and Care Excellence (NICE), a rigorous authority in the psychological field, lists EMDR as a tool for adults grappling with trauma and for children who have not responded to trauma-focused CBT. Yet, some still consider the methods used in EMDR as "alternative," and some researchers continue to debate whether EMDR is more effective than other trauma treatment methods. Dr. Andrew Leeds, author, researcher, and trainer in EMDR, shared in his keynote address at EMDRA 2023 his concern that the view of EMDR from critics has not changed much, and that some researchers are still trying to dismantle the effectiveness of EMDR, claiming there is still "not enough evidence."[6]

EMDR client case examples

Anyone who has experienced trauma, is stressed out (and we all are, including the impact from Covid-19), feels stuck, or finds that "therapy just isn't going anywhere," may benefit from EMDR. Additionally, there are modified, "advanced" versions of EMDR that can be helpful when early attachment figures (parents and other care-givers) were not present, nurturing, consistent, and caring. Leeds (2016) says EMDR has been successfully applied in diverse cultural settings around the world for the treatment of PTSD, cancer, and just dealing with life.[7]

This is an example of when "parts work" (connecting to the inner child, defiant teenager) or the Ego State Theory of EMDR may be helpful (Shapiro 2016): "The more dissociated the client, the more they project, and the more we clinicians feel their pain" (Robin Shapiro, personal communication, January 6, 2023). This is how we can help clients notice they may have "one foot in the present, and the other in the past," when they are so angry, or just can't let that resentment go. This is when the critic section of the cortical brain can step in (yes, the brain stuff again) and the Inner Critic (the Committee, Monkey Mind, inner chat room) starts rambling (could be a protector part) negative sentiments about doing EMDR or even continuing with therapy. Here is where people say, "Shouldn't you be over this by now?" Or, "You are going to a therapist for that?" Or, "I am over this, I am 'done' with therapy"... And, by the way, we are never "done" with taking care of ourselves...

Here is an example of how EMDR can be adapted. There are also more restricted or contained approaches in EMDR that can be used or modified, such as in critical incident debriefing, single episode trauma, or when several presenting stressful problems are brought to the session to address (please get EMDR training to learn how to use this).

EMDR CONTAINED APPROACH

Shannon, an EMDR therapist, shared the following story:

I had a client I stopped seeing in psychotherapy because she met her goals and was getting ready to give birth in a couple of weeks. About three months later, she

---

6   www.youtube.com/watch?v=TLJh5zsib8U
7   www.youtube.com/watch?v=TLJh5zsib8U

returned to me because she had experienced a traumatic birthing experience. The client reported about 5–7 flashbacks a day and an immense amount of guilt and shame. I decided to use EMDR because it was processing the birth and the feelings regarding the experience. When it came time to enter phase 4, we processed the traumatic birthing experience in one session. In the next session, about two weeks later, the client reported that she had not experienced one flashback since we utilized EMDR to process the experience.

Here are several examples of clients with whom I used EMDR (some have provided direct permission; others have been edited to protect their privacy).

PHOBIA

The client is a 37-year-old female whom I will call Cheyenne, who presents herself for EMDR therapy specifically to address her fear of vomit and vomiting. This fear has been present in her life since she was six years old. Cheyenne is married, has two children, works as a mental health therapist, and is trained in yoga instruction. Since she is applying what she learned in her EMDR training, we went right into what she wanted help with using EMDR.

To conceptualize this case, over the first two sessions, stages 1–3 of EMDR were conducted (safety, case conceptualization, preparation and assessment). Because of her work as an EMDR therapist, Cheyenne was familiar with many techniques to self-soothe and regulate emotions. Next, a trauma timeline was created, and the therapist used this as a guideline for the target sequence plan (where to begin). Cheyenne voiced concern about confidentiality and privacy relating to the therapeutic relationship, and I validated this concern and communicated my adherence to ethics and privacy, along with informing Cheyenne that during the course of reprocessing, details of the memories need not be articulated verbally; meaning, I did not need to know all the specifics, unless she wanted to share them with me. Cheyenne seemed comforted knowing this.

We spent four sessions referring back to the target sequence plan and working through stages 4–7 of EMDR (desensitization, installation, body scan, and closure). At the start of each session, Cheyenne identified more negative beliefs she held about herself relating to situations in the past (SUDS: 8) and what she would rather believe about herself then and now (VoC: 2); for example, she chose to work on the negative cognition "I am shameful," which shifted to "I am worthy of love." During each session, I invited Cheyenne to select the issue (the same memory, or a different one if something had shifted between sessions) that she wanted to start with. I then invited her to select a word to identify the issue (then I did not need the details) and to rate on a scale of 0-10 how intense or activated around this issue she felt right now (using SUDS). Examples of the target labels were "school" and "Dad's critical words." During the reprocessing, Cheyenne verbalized her thoughts four-to-five times between sets, but mostly she just nodded and said "Change" in response to the question, "What do you notice now?" to which I would reply, "Go with that." We had established the STOP signal at the beginning of stage 2, so Cheyenne knew she could halt the session at any time if she needed.

During the phase 4 (desensitization) processing, I became aware that other neural networks had opened up: "I am shameful" and "I am bad." I did not know specifically what Cheyenne was working on but felt that she knew, and I "trusted the EMDR process" and just kept going until the SUDS dropped to zero. In the final session, after the body scan and strengthening her preferred belief (VoC: 7), I used the AIP model (the three-pronged approach of imagining past, present, and future situations) for Cheyenne to apply her newly discovered knowledge about herself (adaptive preferred beliefs) in case something came up to trigger what had brought her to me...all were tapped in slowly to strengthen this current and future template. The fear of vomiting was gone.

TRANSFERENCE

Case consultation (supervision) is always recommended when a therapist is wondering whether they are helping or getting in the way of the client's journey. A consultee (a therapist who came to me for guidance and input) shared:

> A few things have come up with one of my clients seeking EMDR and I wondering if I am trying to control the session or is it her. We are using the contained/ restricted processing of EMDR (discussed and informed consent obtained prior to beginning the session). She does not like it when I direct her to a take breath in between BLS sets and is asking for longer sets (more than 15-to-20 passes of BLS). She does not want to do a calm/peaceful place or other resourcing exercises. When we were identifying her negative cognitions, she seemed very resistant, so instead, she asked to just focus on the memory to target (so I "went with that"). This last session, I reminded her that we agreed to process the memory she gave me (single incident); she told me she wanted longer sets, and I was concerned other memories might "pop up." I did feel a little friction throughout the session because of this, and we were able to talk about it at the end of session. I did share that shorter sets are for a reason, etc.

Then the consultee said to me: "I'm curious about your thoughts and how you would go about this." I told her (and other EMDRIA-approved consultants may have different ideas, as "it depends" on many factors) I would go back, do some case conceptualization, and go over the target sequence planning, as the purpose of therapy (what brought her to you) may have shifted. I also suggested she explore how/with whom/when she was trained in EMDR (some trainers emphasize different things during basic EMDR training). And maybe there were some blocking beliefs (see the Blocking Beliefs Questionnaire in Chapter 6) or memories/events/situations (past, present, future) she had never shared with anyone that were "popping up." We also talked about what was coming up for her to doubt what she was doing with this client (if you don't know why you are doing what you are doing with a client, always obtain consultation).

When the consultee returned after her next session with the client, she shared with me that while she was an EMDRIA-approved consultant, she had never experienced EMDR for herself (this was interesting to me, as during basic EMDR training, part of the requirement of the training is that participants are paired off to "practice" what they are learning on each other). She said that she initially came to consult with me because she was feeling a lot of guilt about raising her fees at the end of the year, that her clients would get mad at her if she did. In exploring this further, she identified a moment in her life when this felt similar, especially issues concerning her family. She said things like she felt like she couldn't speak up because she was seen as the "know it all" in the family, or as the "therapist who is always analyzing." (She disclosed she was in therapy, and I suggested she talk to her therapist or seek out an EMDR therapist to help her process this.)

During the consultation, I shared about my training and how I do shorter sets to keep someone within their window of tolerance before doing unrestricted work. I also told her about resourcing and went over what that would look like. She agreed to try all of it, and I reassured her what she was doing was great...that her client kept coming back and telling *her* what *she* needed. This case consultation example demonstrates how important it is to remember how and when clients seek us out, because sometimes things shift.

ANGER AND PTSD

This was shared with me (with permission) by a client named John, a retired New York police officer, who said right away when I recommended EMDR and how it works, "this will never work for me." Here is what he said after experiencing EMDR:

> My rage and verbal outbursts were over the top. I did not think anything was going to help—and of course I was not going to let any of my law enforcement friends know that I was in therapy—you are supposed to just be tough and handle it. Thank God for the psychiatrist I was seeing that sent me to you—who I later stopped seeing!
>
> Using the tappers in EMDR therapy helped me stay laser-focused in session on what was truly bothering me. It allowed me to remove stuff I was thinking about that wasn't good for my mental health. I was able to let go of many resentments. And the breathing exercises really helped me figure out what emotions I was feeling at a particular time. Before I came to therapy and tried EMDR, every emotion I would experience turned directly into anger. By using the breathing techniques you taught me, I was able to figure out my emotions at that particular moment, such as feeling sad, worried, etc.
>
> It all helped me figure out who I am mad at and why. When I used to get angry, I would take it out verbally on my wife. Now when I get angry or mad, the first thing I say to myself is, "why am I mad and who am I mad at?" Within seconds,

I am able to rationally take care of the pending issue. I can't remember the last time my wife and I had an argument.

PREPARING FOR SURGERY

A 42-year-old married woman of Hispanic origin, whom I will call Martina, was referred to me by a cancer center. The referral source said, "I have a client who is having surgery in ten days. Is that enough lead time to do EMDR with her?" I said, "Give me 20 minutes" (a quote from Dr. David Grand, whom you will read about in Chapter 4, the Brainspotting chapter). Luckily, I had a cancellation and was able to see the client the next day. She plopped down on my couch, burst into tears, and told me that she had three young children, one with special needs, and now she was being "forced to" do "another procedure she did not want to do." When I asked what she meant by being "forced again," she said those words immediately took her back to what is referred to in EMDR as the "touchstone memory:" When she was in first grade (age six), her mother took her to have "a procedure that she was forced to have done," which required the medical team to strap her down to use a suppository; her mother left her alone in the room while they did this. As a result, we had to quickly switch gears (yes, informed consent was provided before we started), and we just "went with that" working memory—she was ready!

Martina described the fear and uncertainty about being at the hospital and how her mother had left the room, leaving her alone "with all those people," and she burst into hysterical crying. I said, "Let's go get her!" "Who?" she asked. I said, "Your younger part, little Martina, who is so scared and alone." Then she looked at me and said, "But I have so many questions and fears about *this* surgery." (The cortical brain and her protector parts try to derail the process.) I assured her not to worry, that we would get to that. Using parts work here (an advanced EMDR technique, simplified here), we obtained permission from her younger part to bring her back into the present, where her older, wiser self could protect her and keep her safe. The client sobbed as she told me, "She is here now." I told her to tell her younger part that the earlier experience in the hospital was over and that her older, wiser Martina was here to protect her now. Martina was clutching her heart, sobbing, so I handed her my Raggedy Ann doll (which was on the seat next to her), and said "Here, hold her. And by the way...do you know what it says under her dress?" She shook her head "no," and I showed her the words "I love you."

After she rocked and sobbed with Raggedy Ann (yes, I gave the doll to her), she gazed into my eyes and asked "Am I cured?" I answered: "You might be!" Once she calmed down, we closed the session with her wanting to know why that memory had "popped up out of the blue." I told her it was because the two events were connected—both were procedures she did not want to have happen.

During the second session, we processed the upcoming surgery. But before we started the target for this session, Martina wanted to tell me something. She said: "It was weird, when I left your office, I put Raggedy Ann in the trunk of my car. Then I realized she does not belong there; she belongs in the front seat with me. Now she is always in the car with me." I asked her how that made her feel to have Raggedy Ann with her. She said, "More confident, and that I will be fine." We slowly tapped that in to reinforce it, and then talked about her taking Raggedy Ann to the surgery center if she wanted.

The second session went like this:

- Target for processing: Anticipation of upcoming surgery to put in the port for chemo treatment.

- Negative cognition (NC) she linked with this: "I am permanently damaged. I should have done something to prevent this" (meaning the cancer).

- Preferred cognition (PC) (what she wants to believe): "I am fine the way I am."

- The intense emotions she feels when she thinks about the surgery: "Despair, sick to my stomach."

- SUDS: 10.

- Location in the body where she is feeling all this: "Stomach and chest."

After doing the BLS about ten times, the SUDS went down to a 2. Then she said she wanted to ask me some questions, as she knew I was a breast cancer survivor. I asked her if this meant she was ready to close down the EMDR session. She said she felt much calmer all over and that she would be "fine no matter what." I asked her how true this felt, thinking about the upcoming surgery (based on VoC), and she said a "seven." We "installed this" with slow BLS and the color blue.

To debrief from the session, she asked me if I had had a port put in for the chemo treatments. I told her, "yes," and I showed her my scar (near my left shoulder). She asked me if it hurt. I told her I didn't remember it hurting but was glad I had done it so I did not have to keep getting stuck with needles and hooked up to an IV every time I went for the chemo infusions.

Then she told me horror stories she had heard about people getting burnt by the radiation treatments. I told her I was burnt but it wasn't bad, and asked if she wanted to see the burned area below my breast (she was getting a mastectomy, like me). She said, "Really?" I said, "yes," just to change what she was imaging from the horror stories she had been told. So, I showed her. With an instant sigh of relief and look of calm on her face and she said, "I cannot thank you enough, and can't believe you shared all this with me." I told her I did this for her because, like her, I had been terrified, and someone had done this for me when I was going through all this, so I was "paying it forward." She hugged me, and when she left, said, "I never knew this could be so helpful so fast."

Now some of you may be thinking, "How unprofessional, inappropriate, boundaries not in check." All I can say to you is, unless you have been through a life-changing event like cancer and the invasive, body-altering treatment...you cannot relate. And what I learned in graduate school—if you are sharing something personal—make sure you incorporate "WAIT" (Why Am I Talking)...that you are being authentic and that what you're sharing is in service of the client. I think this worked here. I am grateful for the Cancer Warriors who helped me through the cancer journey (Patty Liebman, LCSW and the Sari Center; Prinster 2014; Zuckweiler 1998).

I called Martina the week after her procedure and asked her how it had gone. She said, "I am fine the way I am. I am myself again, and Raggedy Ann is with me."

RECOVERY AND COPING AFTER "AN ACCIDENT"

Jennifer, aged 50, was referred to me by a plastic surgeon I know, as she had been in an accident. The presenting problem was that she had been brutally attacked by a dog at a place that keeps pets over night when owners are out of town. The pen the dog was in closed behind her, locked, an alarm sounded, and the dog leapt at her, clawing and biting her forearms. As a result, she was having plastic surgery and physical therapy for the injury caused by the dog.

During our EMDR work together, we focused on the image of the dog's teeth (which was causing her nightmares and flashbacks), the sound of the dog growling, and the guilt that she had somehow caused this, as she had not taken extra caution before entering the pen.

In one session, we used tapping to help between sessions if or when she was triggered, for example, by the bark of dogs in the neighborhood or dogs barking on a television show. When triggered, she gets hot flashes and starts sweating. During the talk portion of the session, we discussed her fear of dogs she does not know, and that given what had happened to her, this "anticipatory anxiety" and protective part of her may be a very *normal* response.

- NC for the session: "I am not safe, I am in danger, something is going to happen."

- PC: "I am not in danger; I know how to keep myself safe and feel calm."

- SUDS: 7.

- VoC: 3

- Body location: stomach.

During the BLS, the SUDS went from 7 to 0, and the VoC was strengthened to 7. During debriefing, we reviewed what she could do when she was triggered: She will do a "reality check," look around, and realize, "I can't get attacked by a dog on TV," or "Dogs in the neighborhood are not in my house," and anything else she needs to make sure she feels secure and has no reason to think "something is going to happen."

She ended the session by saying, "This tapping stuff really does work."

My personal experience with EMDR

> *We hate that we don't have control over our (or others') mortality. (Robin Shapiro, personal communication, January 6, 2023)*

Although I was originally trained in EMDR in 2002, I thought it was too "woo woo" and didn't use it in my therapy practice (van den Hout *et al*. 2001). Then, in January 2014, I received a diagnosis of stage 3 breast cancer. As a result, I took the EMDR basic training again and sought out an EMDR therapist to help me navigate the cancer journey and double mastectomy.

When I found out after MRIs, mammograms, etc. that the test results revealed that I had stage 2 breast cancer, I was informed that I would have to have a full mastectomy of the right breast. Just like that, right "out of the blue." Trying to wrap my head around the image of having one breast seemed very weird to me, so I told the surgeon and oncologist to just take them both. This turned out to be a good idea as during surgery it was discovered that there were cancer cells floating around in the left breast anyway, which meant I found out after the double mastectomy I actually had stage 3 breast cancer, and future surgery would have been necessary. The doctors also ended up discovering and removing eight lymph nodes with cancer from the underside of my right arm—the cancer was caught just in time, as it was rapidly and aggressively spreading.

The cancer engaged me in some serious self-reflection. Here I was, a non-smoker, yoga teacher/therapist, certified trauma and addiction professional, licensed somatic psychotherapist utilizing complementary and mindful approaches in my private practice, someone who teaches and writes about these mindbody practices, eats healthy, exercises... "WHY ME?!" Well, why not me? Who was I to be so special to be immune from a disease that is attacking one out of every six women in the United States? Having overcome asthma and being hit by that drunk driver while training for the New York City marathon (which led to The FUN® Program), I knew it was my job to find out the meaning *again*—this time the meaning of being diagnosed with stage 3 breast cancer.

While the supportive therapy and guidance in mental imagery (Epstein and Fedoroff 2012) I was doing was helpful, I was looking for something to help relieve or remove the grief and shock that just seemed stuck in my brainbody. I researched what type of therapy, yoga, and body treatments were recommended specifically for dealing with breast cancer, and while the counselling center I was at did not offer them, I found many references to EMDR and trauma-informed yoga (Schwartz 2016; 2018; 2022). So, I decided to jump in and renew my interest in EMDR certification and go through my own experience of engaging in EMDR therapy for me!

And things really did become released after my first experience in EMDR therapy. The intense emotions about my body becoming deformed from the surgeries and hearing the EMDR therapist actually say, during processing, "I don't know how you are handling it. I could not imagine going through what you are." Now, while we trained EMDR therapists are advised to refrain from commenting while clients are processing, hearing this therapist say this to me was so reassuring. It affirmed that, yes, Kathy, what you are going through is very intense. For me, him sharing this with me, I had that "felt-sense" that he is a very attuned, empathetic, regulated, caring EMDR therapist (I hope you find one like this too!).

But there was more for me to realize as I underwent the cancer journey. Once again, I needed to return to The FUN® Program I had created. I had "forgotten" that The FUN® Program needed to remain in place even when I was not having fun! During this time, my inner chat room said things like: "What about your private practice? Your clients can't see you like this." My initial fear was that my clients would go find another therapist—I mean, who wants a therapist with cancer? I imagined them thinking, "I might catch it [meaning cancer]" Or, "She may die, and then what am I supposed to do?" Or, "I am in the middle of an intense divorce or court case... who wants a bald woman who can't remember things because she has chemo brain?" Or, "I need to see someone several times a week, is she able to do this?" But in the end, most of my clients continued their therapy with me. One even said to me: "Take care of yourself, Dr. Shafer, so you can take of us."

Thankfully, and with a lot of hard work (self-care and therapy), not only did I survive, but I have remained cancer-free. Life has returned to "normal." Since 2017, I regularly use EMDR with clients, and since 2020, I am an EMDRIA-approved consultant and coach, helping EMDR-trained therapists integrate EMDR into their psychotherapy practices and become certified in EMDR.

Then, in 2023, while I was writing this book, my mother died—and I again went back to EMDR and The FUN® Program for myself. The experience of having to abruptly shut down my practice to tend to my mother's failing health and sudden death, the grief that ensued, and the internal issues and questions that arose within me (again!) made it crystal clear that I needed to be intensely practicing what I preached about behavioral health to get through it all again.

I deepened my relationship to yoga (gentle movement or restorative poses), meditation ("no one can control my mind but me"), and breathing exercises ("I need to breathe to be here"). I have also continued being in my own therapy, communicating my needs and showing up—that is what my private practice and life is—role-modeling self-care and expressing what I want/need. According to Weintraub (2004), the yoga mat "itself becomes the place where you show up with your whole self." That is what my office became. So, in my practice where you are supposed to be neutral and have limited self- disclosure, I found it necessary to at least let my current clients know again what was going on in my personal life (my mom's declining health) causing me to cancel appointments and abruptly shut my office down temporarily.

EMDR would also play a critical role for me at this time. In order for you to understand, let me share what happened during that time in more detail.

When my mom's health suddenly started to decline at the age of 93, I shut down my private psychotherapy practice immediately (it sounded like the end was near). Cancelling all appointments and future commitments, I left Florida to be with her in Toledo, Ohio. Three weeks later, she seemed to make a turn. She appeared "fine," alert, and still somewhat independent. Because my mom was to have a medical procedure, my sister Teri came from Florida to be with her so that I could return home to take care of some medical concerns. The day I left, Teri was with my mom, she was sitting in her chair, dressed, and getting ready to go have her hair done. I kissed her good-bye and said I would see her on Mother's Day (within the month). She responded cryptically: "If I make it that far."

My mom seemed to make it through her procedure fine (so did I), and Teri left to go back to her home in Florida. Two days later, on Easter Sunday, my mom called me and said in a slurry voice, "Kathy, they are killing me." The hospice nurse who was with her got on the phone and told me my mom's health was "taking a turn," and they were giving her morphine to make her comfortable. Shocked at the sudden "turn," my sister and I both made plans to go back to Toledo. However, due to weather conditions on the east coast of Florida, it took a week to get back there—shutting down my practice and cancelling everything *again.*

When I landed in Detroit, I phoned my sister, who told me to come straight to my mom's apartment. When I got there, my mom was unresponsive, just lying there, breathing with her mouth open. When I talked to the hospice nurse, she said with a smile, "Knowing your mom's need to be in control, this could go on for a month." That is not what happened.

It sounds "woo-woo" but that night in my hotel room I felt my mom's spirit/energy come right into the room and crawl into bed with me. I sat straight up and could not figure out where I was. When I realized I was in Toledo in a hotel room, I said to myself, "Today is the day." That morning, I went to my mom, and even though she was unresponsive, because I was told that hearing is the last sense to go, I told her, "Mom, I felt you come to me last night, so if you are ready to go, we are here." Then I went out into the hall and burst into tears (I did not want her hear to me cry). I called my partner, Dennis. He said to go back into the room and hold the phone up to her ear, which I did. "Mrs. Shafer," he told her, "Don't worry about Kathy, I am going to take care of her. Now you can go to heaven and see Mr. Shafer, my mom, and others waiting to greet you."

Later that afternoon, my sister and I closed her door to have "the talk" with her. We both told her we loved her, that we would be okay, and that if she was ready to go, we were there. Then we sat on either side of her bed and started fun banter back and forth while looking at silly posts on Facebook. "Mom, look at this, and I know you liked me better than Teri but you were more worried about her because 'she is all by herself'" (a private joke), and we both burst out laughing. Then we looked at our mom. She had stopped breathing. Teri said, "She's gone." What we hope happened is that the last thing she heard was us telling her we loved her and the sound of us laughing on either side of her.

Grief is complicated. Even though there had been a grief lecture in Psychology

101 when we covered the subject of death and dying, there is no way to actually be prepared for the death of a family member, even when we think we are. Robin Shapiro, lead EMDR trainer and an internationally renowned author, helped me work through the "worst part" of my mom's death (for now?), using what is called the "two-handed interweave." The worst part for me was wishing I had stayed in Toledo or wishing my mom had not had the procedure and thinking that it was my fault because I left to get my own procedure done.

Robin directed me to "put" on one hand, "I wish [I had stayed, that mom had not had the procedure, that she wouldn't have died, etc.]" and on the other hand: "It's my fault." Robin then directed me to notice what happened when I went back and forth between these two "parts" of myself. Then she asked me: "Would having stayed, her not having the procedure, not allowing the hospice to do their job, etc.... have made any difference or let her live longer?" This "simple" intervention, which some call "parts" work, helped me feel relief and understand that the good thing to focus on was the time I did spend with my mom, that I had made it back before she died, and that Teri and I were both there to help her exit.

Now what? (Back to the *N* in The FUN® Program)

Obtaining and providing professional or personal support of any kind needs to begin by connecting to the individual while they reclaim control from challenging incidents (in my case, the cancer diagnosis, the chemo treatments, the body dysmorphia, the death of my dog JJ, the death of my father, and then the death of my mother, the despair of the loss of support from significant others). When a person is confronted by such intense and emotional events, the impulse to run, avoid, deny, and minimize rather than confront the impact of the event head on can be too overwhelming. Such avoidance strategies can be behavioral (isolating, overworking, imposed self-neglect, etc.), or addictive (alcohol, drugs, shopping, impulsive eating, etc.), so they need to learn how to process everything in an emotional and physical way that does not cause further impact to themselves or others. These are the recovery goals I set for myself and for working with my clients: to move from reliving and remaining in the trauma/diagnosis/grief to embracing recovery and reinventing who I am and why I am here *now*.

In summary, everyone experiences varying degrees of stress, mood disturbances, and trauma over the life span. However, for some of us, the impact and destructive effects of events never really "end." We now have the skills to help ourselves and our clients work on their recovery/recurrence journey. The integration of EMDR into the clinical session, with some psychoeducation about neuroscience—how memory is stored in the brainbody, helps clients understand, and then be able to "talk" about what happened, and what is still affecting them now.

Shapiro (2009, p.18) says that explaining what happens in EMDR sessions in physical terms can be helpful and "less shaming than other explanations":

Your body has three main nerves that connect to your brain. One turns on to put you in red alert, fight-or-flight mode. One turns on when you're socially or pleasantly engaged. And one is the dimmer switch, slowing down the body's and brain's responses. It sounds like your dimmer switch has been stuck for a long time causing your depression. We're going to work together to turn the light back to full on.

This process of being present while clients share their feelings of sadness, anger, helplessness, fear, and shame expands their window of tolerance. Differentiating the past from the present, along with the consistent, caring relationship with the attuned therapist, supports clients in developing trust—there are actually good, well-intentioned beings out there—and a present awareness of hope for the limitless gifts of the future.

While we are in deep respect and grateful for Shapiro's discovery and creation of the EMDR protocol, we need to remember that we are therapists first (with our own clinical and personal past), and we must always remain client-centered and clinically attuned to the needs of our clients. And please remember, dear therapist, "EMDR is an evidence-based practice and keeping to its fidelity is important. If we don't maintain fidelity, we can quickly find ourselves practicing outsides the bounds of EMDR" (Kase 2023, p.165). When clients ask us anxiously before a session, "Will this work?" according to Remen (1996), we become their "first witness," holding the secure space in the present, "one foot in the peaceful calm office, the other in a world beyond imagination." Even more than our experiences, our beliefs can become our prisons. We now have many ways, including the potent work of EMDR, to become free as we keep falling awake and work to help others do the same.

CHAPTER 3: VOCABULARY AND FOLLOW-UP CONCEPTS

Here are some words and topics about the FUN® approach to EMDR for your further study and reference:

- Affect bridge

- AIP model

- Attachment-focused EMDR

- Back-of-the-Head Scale

- Blocking beliefs

- BLS (bilateral stimulation)

- Body scan

- Case conceptualization

- The CIPOS (Constant Installation of Present Orientation and Safety) Procedure

- Cognitive interweaves

- Connect the Consequences

- The Container

- DeTUR (Desensitization of Triggers and Urges)

- Ego state therapy

- Eight phases of EMDR

- EMD, EMDr, EMDR

- EMDR 2.0

- FSAP (Feeling-State Addiction Protocol)

- Floatback technique

- The Four Elements Exercise

- Go with that...

- Informed consent

- LOUA (Level of Urge to Avoid)

- Loving Eyes Protocol

- Parts work

- The Pendulation Exercise

- Polyvagal-informed EMDR

- Positive Affect Tolerance and Integration protocol (PAT)

- RDI (Resource Development and Installation)

- STOP signal

- SUDS (Subjective Units of Distress Scale)

- Target sequence planning

- TICES (Trigger, Image, Cognition, Emotion, Sensation/SUD, and resulting Behavior)

- VoC (Validity of Cognition scale)

- Window of tolerance

CHAPTER 4

Brainspotting—Where You Look Affects How You Feel

> *The eyes are the interpreters of the soul. (Cicero)*
>
> *I believe the greatest gift I can conceive of having from anyone is to be seen by them, heard by them, and to be understood and touched by them. The greatest gift I can give is to see, hear, understand and to touch another person. When this is done I feel contact has been made. (Satir 1976)*

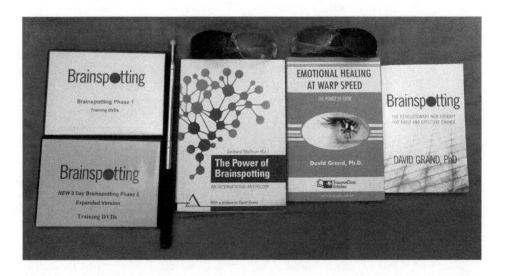

Have you ever noticed when you or a client are talking about or sharing something upsetting or uncomfortable, you/they look away, perhaps in several directions? In terms of body language and eye contact, we have been conditioned to believe that if we are not looking directly at a person, in the eye, and maintaining this eye contact when we are talking to them, we immediately think the person is being rude, avoiding, or may be hiding something (especially if their arms are crossed).

What if, in fact, this is not true—and may be quite the opposite? What if, when we look away, or when our clients soften or change their gaze while expressing what they want to share, and become fixated on a certain visual spot, there may be a lot more going on in the brainbody, at that moment, than we can identify now? (Yes, the brain forest again.) What if, by noticing where our clients look and encouraging them to keep their gaze and to focus their eyes when they feel most activated while talking instead of looking directly at us, that this may, in fact, be more welcoming, inviting, relieving, and helpful for *them*?

The origins of Brainspotting

The core of Brainspotting (BSP) is the attunement of the regulated therapist, who is watching where the client is looking, helping them notice activation of sensations in the body, embracing what is referred to as the uncertainty principle, and finding "the spot," sometimes with the aid of a pointer, where things seem or feel most activated (intense). This means that once the brainspot is determined (by the client and therapist together), the client accesses and reveals traumatic memories and intense emotional situations, all while resetting the nervous system so regulation can occur— no matter what happens or is revealed in the BSP session. Huh? Meaning that during a BSP session, this mindful, secure, focused attention for accessing information to process occurs when the client and therapist together find the activated network... the brainspot(s) in the client's visual field, which is often "held" by a pointer.

Discovering and establishing the most activated eye positions with the pointer (from eye blinks, body twitches, etc.) happens between the client and therapist so the brain can access and reveal information from the past, present, or future concerns (like watching a movie) to let us "see" what is important to be discussed and "go from there." When a person is nervous or anxious, or when there are no words to describe and express what has them activated (anxious, angry, sad, feeling hopeless, etc.), or when we are "not sure where to begin," we may find ourselves looking to the left, the right, up, or down, trying to figure out what to say. How about, instead of "assuming" that when people are not making eye contact or looking at us it is because they are "avoiding" or "hiding" something, we consider that what may in fact be happening is that they are searching for what Grand called the "brainspot" (using a variety of ways to determine and access this). This activated brainspot, determined with assistance from the entry point of the retina (or the other senses), engages specific areas in the subcortical brain where information, history, and details about everything all at once are waiting to be located and accessed. What if this "brainspot," as Grand discovered, actually opens the curious subcortical, neurological brainstem door to help all the other nervous systems and neural pathways light up and "speak," to help us determine what in fact we want or need, or find the words to say?

This is what Grand noticed and became "curious" about, leading to his creation of the integrative healing model he calls Brainspotting. In BSP, the therapist creates the neurobiological frame by finding the resonant eye positions with the client, who is activated around their issue of choice. The therapist then guides the client to maintain their focus on the spot and mindfully observe their inner process, step by step. The therapist then tracks the client's processing closely, yet openly, wherever it goes. This attuned, witnessing presence provides the relational frame known in other therapies as the *holding environment*. In BSP, this relational frame is continually focused on by the therapist and client attending to the brainspot, the body sensations, and the processing (Grand 2013; Grand and Goldberg 2011; Wolfrum 2021). Originally "discovering" and creating BSP in 2003 during his work with professional performers and athletes, Grand found that determining the relevant activated eye position(s), using a variety of what he calls "setups," torpedoes sensory information to the subcortical brain to access and erupt intense emotions, memories, or issues. These neurological brainbody mechanics during BSP bring all this information to conscious cortical awareness for processing during the session.

Grand discovered that where the eyes look—holding "the frame" of the identified brainspot(s) location—provides deep access for information/data stored in the regions of the subcortical brain (the brainstem and spinal cord). In other words, "where you look affects how you feel." Western therapies have not considered the importance of accessing these deeper regions of the brain that cannot be reached by traditional talk therapy or mainstream psychotherapy. This is because cognitive behavioral therapy (CBT) has nothing to do with understanding the central nervous system! Or, in fact, what is going on in our brain or physical body when we are traumatized or feeling stressed out! We don't say to ourselves "Oh, oh, I need to engage my vagal brake and be more ventral" (back to Chapter 1, the brain chapter) (Dana 2021) (as stated earlier, our educational systems do not teach us anatomy and neurology or how these systems work). Therefore, finding the brainspot via the relevant eye position(s) can directly bypass the protective, defensive, critical, and analytical cortical prefrontal cortex—the type of processing that occurs during traditional talk therapy. According to Grand (direct communication, May 19, 2023), anxiety, panic, and flashbacks are clues that developmental traumas are present and stored in the brainbody. Finding the activated brainspot(s) enables the whole body's nervous systems to switch on so all its neural sensors can "speak," be "heard," and be recalibrated (reset and relax).

The process of BSP begins by determining the focus and informed consent for the session—in other words, what is going to be "opened up" from the brainspot. Once this is determined the client is asked about how activated they are right now about this issue on a scale from 0–10 (0 = not activated at all to 10 = very activated), and where they feel this in their body (physical sensation). The fixed eye position (the brainspot) is then discovered from watching the client's eyes (blinking) and facial gestures, and noting where the pointer or eyes need to stop and focus to secure in place the intense physical sensation of the "brainspot." The brainspot(s) are located together with the therapist and held in place for the client, usually with the use of a pointer, to help the client maintain the focused gaze. Then the therapist WAITs (remember this acronym?—Why Am I Talking?) and the silence (what Grand calls "staying in the tail of the comet") enables the client to access and reveal what is going on—all by focusing on the brainspot—and the only talking that occurs is from the client (unless the therapist asks if there is any information/facts/emotions they wish to express) regarding what insights they are having—if they want to.

The activation and revelations that can occur in BSP can be extremely helpful when there may be no words (sometimes silence says much more) to describe what is going on when we are upset, or to gain insight and make connections about why this intense state of reaction is happening now or does not seem to be getting any better. Grand explains that survivors of developmental trauma often go into what he refers to as "compliance mode" during the therapy session, which we need to be aware of and prevent (direct communication, May 19, 2023). This can happen when emotions or the memories accessed are too intense, and the client may instead try to shut down (vagal brake) if they think the therapist does not want to hear about it or get the impression they are not "doing it right" (the therapy). Sometimes intense memories or emotions keep coming up instead of going away—because *healing takes time.*

BSP is designed as a therapeutic tool that can be integrated into many healing modalities and other forms of psychotherapy. According to Grand, sometimes the speed of the eye movements that can occur in EMDR may be too activating. Grand describes BSP as a relational resource model—meaning, at the activated brainspot, deep somatic neural processing uncovers memories like scenes in a movie. While this is happening, the client may be simultaneously sharing the scenes of this "memory movie" they are witnessing with the caring, attuned therapist, who remains quiet. The therapist refrains from engaging or asking questions so that the cortical brain doesn't get activated and the therapist remains in the "tail of the comet" (following the client's lead). This relational attunement expands a client's window of tolerance—embracing the uncertainty principle—that we don't know why things are happening or feeling better, just that they are. This is how healing happens in BSP.

BSP provides another way of letting the client lead the way for the focus and direction of the therapy session. While holding this spot with the pointer, the client can talk if they want to (or not) to let the BSP practitioner know what is going on and what they are experiencing (including whether things are getting more or less intense emotionally and/or what body sensations they are having).

Grand theorizes that this brainbody data is taken in from the external world by what we see, starting with the retina and the five senses (smell, taste, sight, sound, touch). This activating healing process is thought to begin at the agranular cortex (right behind the eyes), and then travels neurologically via the superhighway of the agranular cingulate cortex pathway to the superior colliculus located in the subcortical limbic brain (yes, we are back to brain basics). It is believed that when starting with a brainspot, more detailed "curious" related revelations come into awareness other than just those from the reactive dysregulation alarm center of the amygdala and other regions of the central and autonomic nervous systems.

Once the intensity and the connecting of events (some related and some not) and memories are shared by accessing other neural networks via the brainspot, the more regulated information (from the hippocampus filing cabinet) goes to the corpus callosum. The corpus callosum connects the left and right cerebral hemispheres, going back up the staircase to the prefrontal cortex, where things are making sense *now* to the curious left cortical brain. The talking, thinking analytical cortical brain is not designed to regulate; it does not know how to calm down. Its function is to react (not mindfully respond or adapt) to the information provided from the overactivated amygdala and other regions of the limbic brain. Hence, accessing the information that is blocked from awareness, revealing intense memories and information held in the subcortical brain via the brainspot, is when eruption, release, and regulation happens. Then all that was revealed can be discussed calmly and cortically. (Whew!)

It is only more recently that Grand has coined BSP a "neuroexperiential resource model." This has evolved from his clinical experience and that of the therapists he has mentored through Brainspotting International,which offers training in BSP to healthcare providers around the globe. There are now 125 trainers around the world doing pioneering work for BSP. Grand and his colleagues have found that engaging the subcortical limbic regions of the brainbody initiates regulation, which occurs by accessing the brainspot. Embracing what Grand calls the uncertainty principle, the physical and sensory awareness and self-regulation that occurs in BSP, engages organically and uniquely with each individual and the attuned therapist (Salvador 2021).

Transforming the psychotherapy session

In phase 4 of his BSP trainings, Grand uses BSP to process dreams. In an email prior to a live webinar I registered for on how BSP can work with processing dreams, Grand asked for volunteers to demonstrate how it works. I had a nightmare the night before receiving this email, in which I was watching myself get brutally attacked—like I was getting murdered. I believe this disturbing dream was influenced from a detailed news report about a boy who had disappeared one night in West Palm Beach (near where I live) when he went out to ride his bike and never came home. (He was found dead, killed under an underpass near the interstate.) Grand picked the dream I submitted to be his demo for the BSP training. Not realizing I would be revealing myself and my dream in front of hundreds of people from around the world (one of my core issues is around being seen), I jumped at this learning opportunity.

During my report about the dream, I kept emphasizing how strongly I felt that I knew, that I had "the evidence," of who was responsible for the attack, and that no one was listening to me all while I watched myself get attacked. During the webinar demo, Grand helped me to find my brainspot on my own (looking around my office since we were doing this training with him virtually). He asked me to "go back" into the part of the dream where I felt I needed more answers about why I was being attacked and why I would want to watch this. While holding this spot, what came to me subcortically was that I have the power to protect myself, even when no one is listening. I can take myself out of harm's way. This all happened very quickly. I later shared with a colleague that other things had also become very apparent to me in that moment, but that I did not want to share my private world internationally on Zoom in a live webinar that was being recorded! I also now believe that the rapid connections I was making with Grand on the live webinar was the comfort of knowing that I would have helpful private discussions about everything that came up in my own BSP session with my BSP therapist later that week (it is so, sooooo important that we do our own work if we really want to learn about what we are doing and be helpful to our clients).

Modern and contemporary mental health treatment, Grand contends, is still operating, explicitly and implicitly, from outdated, incongruent language and concepts from our compliance-driven Western medical system. This system continues to view having a mental disorder or a diagnosis in a judgmental, blame-shifting, disabling, "taboo" way, often shaming us and others from seeking help. In the United States and other medical communities around the world, it is implied that trauma-wound manifestations are derived from the cruelties that befall the young and the vulnerable, which excludes the impact of generational trauma, racism, sexism, agism, bullying, and being exposed to angry, mean people. Traditional psychotherapy currently still uses a cognitive-behavioral approach and with its limited, focused- "frame" or "lens" model, often concludes and treats difficulties or "problems" that clients are reporting as faulty mental cognitions or negative thinking. Therefore, according to this mainstream approach, these mistakes in thinking are what need to be corrected in psychotherapy (CBT), and then all will be "fine." Again, exploring and inquiring about how the mechanics of the anatomy and the neurology of the brainbody systems interface thus creating these "stories"—due to trauma, illness, or stress—is ignored.

The entire process of talk therapy as we know it is conducted on a conscious level, usually focusing on current issues and often leaving out important information from the person's history, beliefs derived from past experiences, and stories created from them, even though, as we have seen, somehow the past is still present. Or sometimes a client stops coming to therapy for "not wanting to go there" or saying, "the therapist keeps wanting me to talk about the past and I don't want to." These old concepts and verbiage collide with the language employed in BSP sessions and training: uncertainty, frames, WAIT, "tail of the comet," attunement, presence, body awareness, neurobiology, relevant eye positions, focused mindfulness, dysregulation to regulation, "squeeze the lemon," expansion, staying curious, and attachment disruption, to highlight just a few. Using the methods employed in BSP, understanding the impact of developmental trauma and the role of survival/adaptive dissociation responses neurologically, is what makes BSP a paradigm shift in processing memories and adverse events in the history of our clients. The current language and methods of our mental health fields hardly relate to what we see, know, and do in BSP.

Emotions, Grand says, are rooted in such states as primal fear, rage, and distrust deriving from the fight, flight, freeze, or faint response, or feeling unlovable or invisible, deriving from core attachments. While trauma can make us feel isolated and lonely, in truth we are all in this together. According to Conti (2023), compassion, community, and humanity are intertwined with the full expression of who we are as humans. These can also be in combination with experiences of feeling loved, gratitude, and the joy life can bring us, reflecting the expansive possibility of our quadrillions of synaptic connections. Trauma can hide in all these experiences, often disguised in ways to appear and feel "normal." According to his 2021 keynote address at the second live international BSP conference, Grand emphasized the intuitive (what we think we know) is what we know simply because we know it. It derives from our instinctual animal heritage, a guide for how to survive and thrive in our dynamic, unpredictable environments. In BSP, he says, we are taught to devote most of our efforts to bypassing the neocortex and not get bogged down in the language, thoughts that play no role in regulation. There is, however, a clear place for the neocortical in the experiential aspect of BSP. Frontloading and backloading information are meant to engage the neocortex in anticipating before, and reviewing after, the process that is bookmarked in between. The parting question to the client—"What's your takeaway from this session?"—guides their neocortex to reflect, and then continue reviewing the ensuing post-session processing (brain psychoeducation again).

BSP is open, curious, and respectful of the ideas and practices of others. Grand invites those in the BSP community who possess knowledge of Eastern and Indigenous wisdom and practices to contribute to and build on the neuroexperiential model. Encouraging collective wisdom and "following the tail of the comet together," he hopes to continue building on this integrative resource model of brain-based healing wherever it ventures.

It is the "felt sense" of dysregulation that is the genesis of the client's journey towards pursuing healing. If the dysregulation is painful, disruptive, inhibiting, and continues long enough, the client may be more motivated to take the courageous steps into the healing process. As we greet and welcome a client with attunement, we listen openly, intently, and remain curious. As they spontaneously reveal their story, the client is gently extending their frame (their movie scene from life) out to us "to see it as we receive it." Grand states that we then hold their frame with them and develop it together. By doing so, we are creating with them a secure space that enables them to innately and intuitively move from dysregulation to regulation, not in a step-by-step process, but in a series of unpredictable spirals that mirror the neural processes of exploring and expressing. This is why he calls it, "embracing the uncertainty principle."

In terms of brain activity, during BSP—sometimes called fast-track therapy by Grand—we find the spot(s) by watching where the eyes get locked via the visual pathway from the retina to the superior colliculus in the brainstem via the retinal collicular pathway (the optic nerve/first responder for orienting to the brainspot), which engages the pons, and medulla, at the brainstem where the vagus nerve and central nervous activation (central nervous system) occurs (pain/anticipatory/fight, flight, or freeze/faint). The visceral and tactile sensations in the body from finding the brainspot(s) become the lens through which a person experiences the words, emotions, physical sensations, imagery, and memories to describe what is going on. We learn in BSP trainings that traumas are held in capsules in the brain. These frozen-in-time capsules fire their own signals when triggered and are accessed to process trauma from the information downloaded from the brainspot. Theses trauma capsules can also be accessed by using bilateral sounds or music (the client wears headphones during session) to hold the frame during activation. For example, complex trauma survivors benefit from the use of bilateral sounds to help them remain calmer to process what was "heard" at the time (gun shots, voices/yelling, doors slamming, glass breaking, people laughing, sirens, screaming). At the brainspot, it is believed we are looking directly at the memories through the aid of the retina.

Grand states:

> The Neuroexperiential Model of BSP presents coherent conceptualizations and reflective language for what we know, observe, and do as Brainspotting frame holders. It doesn't reject the current and historical psychological and psychotherapeutic models of theory and practice; it builds on and expands beyond them. The Neuroexperiential Model presents a mindful, expansive, inclusive, dynamic, evolving, permeable frame that adjusts to fit the healing needs of those who are drawn to us. The neuro reflects an open, seeking, organic, culturally attuned and respectful model of the nervous system integrated into brainbody systems. The experiential expresses the unity of our conscious awareness, our internal and external environments, and their constant interplay. The Neuroexperiential Model of BSP helps us determine who we are, what we are, where we have been and where we are going. (2021)

In his concluding remarks at the international conference, Grand quoted the Greek philosopher Heraclitus: "No man steps in the same river twice, for it's not the same river and he's not the same man." We are always in process, whether inside the BSP frame or inside the cosmic frame. The BSP session is a snapshot of the moment, a compilation attempting to capture the moving narrative of human existence. The destination (where we end up in the session) is always unknown because there is no destination. Healing is a process, and an expansive one at that.

A Brainspotting session

There are eight stages to a BSP session:

1. Choose the issue to work on.

2. Check on activation—what are the emotions? Determine how intense these are right now with a Subjective Unit of Distress Scale (SUDS) rating (0–10).

3. Identify where these are felt in the body.

4. Locate the eye position (with the pointer or by letting the eyes find the "spot") or place where they feel most activated—the brainspot.

5. Bring in focused mindfulness (welcome in all sensations), access and allow all that is there to come into conscious awareness while we WAIT.

6. Go back to the beginning to assess change or insights made.

7. "Squeeze the lemon" (check to see if there is more activation to be released).

8. Shut the session down and debrief.

Similar to establishing the "presenting issue" in other therapy modalities, BSP therapists determining "the setup" for the BSP session begin with an invitation to the client: "What would you like to work on or open up today?" Grand states that this is another way of asking, "What neuroexperiential frame have you brought into today's session?" Kind of like, what part of your brain would you like to explore today, and how does your neurological system feel about that?

This is why BSP practitioners don't immediately ask for an extensive history, collecting details or client impressions. Rather, once the topic for the session is determined, the therapist asks, "How activated are you around this issue?" and "Would you like to open this up?" The "activation" inquiry is mindfully used here because it is a frank, neuroexperiential term neutrally inquiring about nervous system intensity while steering clear of the meaning and explanations of the thinking cortical brain. There is no "too much" or "not enough" activation for the BSP session, as it is what it should be within the client's presentation, tolerance, and consent. If the activation is low and the client appears stable, we may encourage them to challenge themselves by perhaps by inquiring "What upsets you most about this?"—a sort of initial "squeezing of the lemon" (another BSP term)—a mental and courageous jump in and see what they are willing and able to process.

Whatever the level of activation is, the BSP therapist begins there and moves ahead to taking the SUDS (presented earlier and used in EMDR), rating the intensity from 0 to 10. This rating process numerically engages the neocortical aspect of the conscious experiential. Despite being subjective, the SUDS provides a numerical assessment that can be revisited throughout, or at the conclusion of, the session (also done in EMDR). If, during the processing, the SUDS rises, it does not indicate a problem; rather, it may be pointing to dissociative barriers (parts) that are protecting unprocessed trauma. This elevation of the SUDS actually reflects that the process is working by finding its way to and into trauma buried deep in the subcortical regions of the brain.

After obtaining the SUDS, the client is asked, "Where do you feel the activation in your body right now?" This is a purely neuroexperiential question, without any psychological explanation. Grand states that it is like a medical doctor asking a patient, "Where does it hurt?" We accept whatever the client reports, as they know their system best. As the client is observing the activation in their body, their visual systems are simultaneously responding with facial expressions and eye reflexes orienting for a spontaneous brainspot, all being closely observed and watched by the attuned and regulated BSP therapist. BSP therapists quickly move to harness these ocular phenomena, with or without a pointer.

Every person has a unique reaction and experience with BSP. They may even feel awkward "just looking at a spot," since people are conditioned to talk. Just cue them back to the body part where they reported sensation, take another SUDS (0–10) and go from there. Sometimes there is more than one "brainspot" and you can ask them if the activation spot changed when you notice the eyes moving or glancing to another location. Most people will tell you a lot of information just by finding "the spot" and others may say they feel "nothing," in which case, we say, "Notice that you feel nothing and go from there." (They may want to return to cortical processing as this brain therapy is so new to them.)

At the end of a BSP session, clients will frequently say something like, "I have no idea what happened here today, but it was amazing, worked fast, and felt right." Despite the client's conscious participation, it may well be that they are simultaneously noticing internally discharged reflexes that are not observable to the therapist. For example, the client may report feeling sweaty or hot, notice some muscles tightening or twitching, or experience a sudden emotional disturbance or pain intensification, which are all reflexive expressions from the brainstem and spine. Clients may also report the experience of an intense flow of memories, emotions, and associations, all without much verbal exchange—like watching scenes from the movie of their life.

This pragmatic and dynamic shift of memory processing is why some health practitioners consider BSP an alternative form of the bilateral processing that occurs in EMDR. Additionally, embracing the concept of WAIT (Why Am I Talking?) is similar to holding a talking stick, as is done in some Indigenous communities: the pointer or talking stick "secures" the spot and space for what rises, so that the speaker can say what needs to be said and released without interruption. In BSP, we may consider the client as "holding the talking stick" and given respect to "have the floor" with the permission to be heard without judgment or interruption.

Research is now forthcoming on how BSP, along with the other brain therapies I am referring to in this book, is now among the evidence-based practices used to reduce the symptoms associated with PTSD (Horton *et al.* 2024).

PSYCHOSIS

Eve is a 20-year-old female referred to me by her psychiatrist after she was discharged from an involuntary admission to an inpatient psychiatric unit for yet another suicide attempt (she had jumped from the balcony of her parents' condo). She was confined to a wheelchair, and we held sessions virtually via Zoom. She had been diagnosed with psychosis (schizoaffective disorder, nonspecific) and shared with me that she felt she never "got anything" from the therapy or therapists she had previously seen. She also presented with trouble controlling her binge eating, had difficulty providing details about the activities of her daily life, and did not want to follow through with the recommended higher levels of care (such as an intensive outpatient therapy program) where she could be seen more often, be involved in a daily routine, not be so isolated, and meet more people her age.

Given the lack of information about what kind of therapy she was in previously or anything that had been helpful for her, I introduced her to BSP. After our first session, her mother became so curious about the change in her daughter's demeanor and interaction with the family that she asked for a BSP session for herself to understand how it worked and helped someone who had been diagnosed with psychosis—everyone else had "given up on her."

I met with Eve weekly, and we set treatment goals for her daily life activities, boundaries with binge eating, and created professional and education goals. She began to walk (after the injuries from her jump had healed) and she participated in sessions live at my office. Eve's psychiatrist even called and said, "Whatever you are doing with that Brainspotting, keep doing it...the change in her is remarkable."

This client provides a clear example of trusting the uncertainty principle. Sometimes the traditional therapy methods typically used to work with "difficult cases"—for example, those with a history of psychosis or dissociation—may not be helpful. Using BSP succeeded where talk therapy and other approaches hadn't and led to changes creating connections (inner and interpersonal) and perhaps neurological, or energetic, repair.

THE NEED FOR BOUNDARIES

A 33-year-old Orthodox Jewish woman I shall call Helen was referred to me for EMDR therapy. She married at the age of 19 and has four children aged 6 to 12. At the first session, Helen reported that her husband wanted sex on demand and she was embarrassed that she was not being "a good Jewish woman," since the rabbi told her to work on her marriage and be a "good Jewish wife." During the course of our work (weekly, for 10 months) I introduced her to BSP. She began requesting it as she liked the ability to find the spot(s) that was disturbing and could process what was going on without sharing too much detail. After several BSP sessions Helen was able to gain the confidence to go back to the rabbi and let him know that she did not feel her husband was making any progress with his obsessive-compulsive disorder (he had been seeing a different therapist for years) and asked the rabbi's help in finding her husband another therapist. This gain in confidence—asking for what she wanted and setting boundaries with her husband—helped her process. She stopped feeling nauseous during the BSP sessions and moved from feeling trapped to having things she could do when emotionally overwhelmed and triggered. Helen is now feeling that she has worked through stressful situations and is doing the best she can, given her circumstances. (Now the therapist that referred her to me is my client...the miracle of BSP spreads quickly...)

Providing Helen with the choice to experience and choose the treatment approach for her sessions helped her feel empowered and heard, and supported her in realizing that she did have choices in her marriage, family, and personal life, and that this did not conflict with her faith and her role as a married Orthodox Jewish woman. Helen now reaches out to me when she feels she needs a "tune up."

GRIEF WORK USING GAZESPOTTING (NO POINTER NECESSARY)

Stephen, age 30, just lost his younger brother to a rare form of cancer. Stephen and his brother had lived, worked, and shared a lot of time together. He did not trust therapists and had walked out of the session with the last one he had seen. Stephen said, "She was weird, and just sat behind her desk." His family, friends, and the referral source were concerned as he had not shared his grief with anyone, and they worried about how he was coping. After meeting with his parents and family, Stephen brought his "other family" (his close personal friends) to meet me and see if I was "okay/cool." My certified emotional support dog Bentley was there for this one, and I invited them all into the yoga room to give them the choice to sit in a chair or on a cushion or yoga bolster. After the third meeting Stephen agreed to meet with me alone.

As he was sitting in the chair (his choice) his leg began to throb up and down and he said "I don't know if I am ready for this. I was supposed to go first, I am the older brother." I asked him if he wanted to try something and that he would not have to talk much. He said, "Sure," and I showed him the pointer. He looked at me like "What is that?" and I told him I would explain later as it looked like he was really activated and ready to release emotions. Then I asked him how intense all this felt to him now, from 0–10. He said a 10 and that he felt this in his heart. When we found the spot where it seemed most intense by his eyes, and his leg started shaking. I said, "Just notice you are not sure if you are ready for this—and go with that." Then all the crying and emotions just came out about his brother's death. I watched his eyes, and when he was particularly emotional, the "gazespot" appeared (his eyes were locked on one spot in my office). I suggested he just let his eyes stay right where they were and allow what was coming up to come up. And then I practiced WAIT...and let the BSP gazespot do the work.

Since the subcortical brain had been accessed, there were no words that needed to be to be said from my end (so I utilized WAIT). Stephen would just look at me directly, and then go to another brain gazespot around the office. When he said, "I don't have anything else right now," I told him to take a breath and let it go...and asked, "What do you notice now?" And we kept going and I watched him hold his various brainspots.

Near the end of the session I asked him, "What are you learning from all this about yourself? What is helping you right now?" and he said, "This is going to take some time, but I feel calmer"... I asked: "And where do you feel calmer in your body?" And he pointed to his chest...and I said, "Just focus on feeling calmer there right now and give yourself permission to feel calmer."

At this point his leg stopped throbbing and he asked if he could just get up and walk around my office... I said "Of course...please move, get a drink of water, whatever you need." He thanked me and at the next session he told me when he left my office that he had taken a long drive and gone to the beach to walk and talk to his younger brother, who he would someday see again in heaven...

I resourced myself when he left. Self-regulation care is for me, too!

Introducing Brainspotting to your clients

You and your clients are used to how you work in session and that is perfectly okay! If you want to integrate BSP into your practice, start small. Try this little self-spotting exercise (yourself or with a client):

SELF-SPOTTING

- Notice what's on your mind (note the activation on a scale of 0–10, where 0 = neutral or no activation to 10 = highest level of activation, and where you feel it in your body).

- Now look to the right, center, and the left. Find the spot with the most activation and stay there (5 minutes).

- Just see where that goes. Give this some time and space and see what happens.

- Afterwards, notice if you are calmer, grounded, somewhat better, or neutral (take a SUDS, 0–10).

Remember, in BSP we embrace the uncertainty principle (staying in the "tail of the comet"—the client leads us). All we have to go on is the frame—the client's view of what happened (past, present, future) and what to work on.

You may want to explain to your client how BSP works, that holding "the brainspot" (eye gaze) with the steady pointer helps move a person from dysregulation to regulation. During this process, it is thought that what neurosensory messages need to come to the prefrontal cortex are revealed and released. As the therapist and client sit in uncertainty (not sure where it will lead or what will be released) the process that organically occurs in the brain leads the way, referring to following in the "tail of the comet."

You can also share some of the basics of how a session works, including:

- Physical position: BSP is typically a seated practice, where the body is comfortable, yet upright and alert.

- The issue: A current stressor or critical incident in the present, or a past trauma, is being reexperienced because of recent events that are causing the client to engage the fight, flight, freeze, or freeze response.

- Attention: Once the issue has been determined for the BSP session, the client consciously determines with the eye gaze where they feel is the most intense "spot" (where the emotions they have described and the sensations they feel in their body become most intense). The client then places their attention on the "brainspot" (with or without the pointer) and the therapist simply instructs the client to see what happens as they look at this spot and "go from there."

You can also introduce BSP by simply commenting on where a client is looking (the brainspot of eye gaze) while they are talking about something they are working on. You may make a comment like, "When you are remembering the accident/argument/bad dream, I notice that your eyes go over there [tell them what you are witnessing]." Then ask if they would like to open this up further with BSP (although always obtain informed consent).

I also invite my clients to watch YouTube videos about BSP and interviews with Grand to learn more about how the retina of the eye takes us to the exact spot of the brain where the information will be accessed and brought to consciousness without us having to talk very much. We let the brain and body access the neurological systems, no matter what the age, to provide us with all the information—and do the work for us (Baumann 2020).

Falling and staying awake in the subcortical brain

BSP may be used for any number of things: to increase sports performance (where Grand "discovered" it), or to treat body image issues, for trauma relief, for chronic pain, when "there are no words," or for insights not obtained in talk therapies.

Remember, "where you look affects how you feel." So, if you have a session where a client is reporting something happy or a fun experience (or if you want to open up the neural networks to disrupt the looping of negativity), have them find the gratitude or happy FUN® spot (Brown 2015). When I was in Ohio to take care of my mom before she died, I met up with some friends from high school (we all went to DeVilbiss High School, and my mom herself was a DeVilbiss Tiger from the Class of '47). Every time we got together, we laughed, recalled old times, and talked about the dysfunction in our families. So, when I get upset or feel lonely, I think about these times together (there have been many) and allow my eyes (open or closed) to find the spot as I notice and sense the loving feeling in my heart.

Fear, doubt, and trust cannot exist at the same time. Neither can positive and negative beliefs. CBT, BSP, EMDR, and Yoga Nidra all help clients remember what they can do and have done to be resilient—instead of what they cannot do or what happened. Instead of just trying to "forget about it," these brain therapies access the subcortical limbic regions to provide relevant insights into what the client can focus on instead. This mental strength training can be used when doubt, boredom, shame, or depression returns (known as triggers or an emotional relapse). This goes back to the power of intention or focusing discussed earlier: What do you want?

In a recent interview (2022), famous Rock and Roll Hall of Fame recipient Bruce Springsteen told Howard Stern that when you write a song, first you write the lyrics and the music comes later. So, maybe the F of The FUN® Program, the relevant eye in BSP, "going with that" in EMDR, and just lying still in Yoga Nidra are all correct. If we trust that the brain and body can heal themselves, if we just pay attention and do not fall asleep, we may have everything that we need to motivate us to stay awake. We do have the power.

CHAPTER 4: VOCABULARY AND FOLLOW-UP CONCEPTS

Here are some words and topics about Brainspotting for your further study and reference:

- Activation
- Bilateral sound
- Body resource setup
- Dual attunement
- Establishing relevant eye positions
- Expansion
- Go from there
- Guidelines for setting up the frame
- Limbic countertransference
- Narrowing the frame
- Neuroexperiential model
- One-eyed spotting/goggles
- Outside/inside window/rolling/gazespotting
- Pointer
- Regulate the dysregulation
- Resource model
- Shades up/down
- Somatic therapy
- Squeeze the lemon
- Staying curious, connected, compassionate
- Staying in the "tail of the comet"
- SUDS (Subjective Units of Disturbance Scale)
- Superior colliculus
- Uncertainty principle
- WAIT (Why Am I Talking?)
- Where you look affects how you feel
- Window of tolerance
- X-Y-Z axis

CHAPTER 5

Yoga Nidra—Relaxation Is the Challenge, Falling Awake Is the Answer

> *The more we rest as who we are, the less we are at the effect of what is passing through. We can be at peace and steady in the midst of external and internal disturbance. (Desai 2017, p.6)*

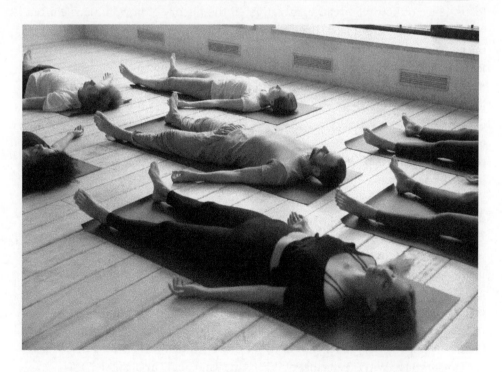

As we continue to explore the brain forest, we are about to travel and step onto a path that may be avoided because it is very misunderstood. For example, when you hear or see that a Yoga Nidra class is being offered at the local gym, yoga studio, or retreat center, what image immediately comes to mind? Please know that the practice of Yoga Nidra does not involve any of the yoga poses typically associated with yoga. You will not be asked to stand on your head, do sun salutations, sit in contorted positions, learn how to do downward facing dog and stay there forever, speak in Sanskrit, worship deities, or give up your religion. Yoga Nidra is deceptively "simple" and is one of the least known and most under-appreciated practices of yoga, yet its mental and physical health benefits are immense (Desai 2017).

To experience Yoga Nidra all you have to do is show up, lie or sit down, and not move for about 40 minutes (with no talking required!). We all need to calm the f*** down (remember the *F* in The FUN® Program in Chapter 2). Yoga Nidra is a tool to stop *doing* and relax...just lie down on a yoga mat or sit in a chair and recharge your brainbody in whatever time you have available. Judith Lasater (2007), the queen of restorative yoga (meaning lying down in class with yoga props to relax deeply) states that the antidote to stress is deep relaxation, which is different from sleep. Among the first to study the benefits of relaxation was Dr. Edmond Jacobson. In 1934 he wrote *You Must Relax*, noting the health benefits of progressive relaxation techniques, which you will learn about in the practice of Yoga Nidra (Jacobson 1962). Then Dr. Herbert Benson (1975), in another first in the study of the impact of stress, coined the phrase the "relaxation response" while studying how yogis in India calm their heart rate while meditating. James Nestor (2020), in his writings about the lost science of how we breathe, investigated the history of how humans shifted from the natural state of nasal breathing to chronic mouth breathing. He references the curiosity researchers had at the Menninger Clinic in 1970, studying how Swami Rama's (from the Himalayas) breathing practices (called pranayama in the science of yoga) calmed his heart rate and slowed his brainwaves to low delta, which is identified with deep sleep. Even though he was so relaxed and ended up snoring during this demonstration, when he "woke up" he was able to provide details of the conversation researchers were having in the room while he was in this place of deep rest. He described and called what he experienced "yogic sleep," a state in which the mind was active while the brain slept.

According to Walker (2017), surveys conducted in 1942 reported only 8 percent of people in the United States slept six hours or less per night; now it is 25 percent. He says this sleep deprivation continues to be encouraged in our work "culture" even though employee health and human resource trainings promote the opposite. These include policies regarding smoking, substance misuse, ethical behavior, and safety, and yet, the mentality of insufficient rest is commonly tolerated and expected. Many cultures and countries understand and condone the need for rest and taking a break or pause. What happened to taking naps (a siesta) or keeping the stores closed on Sunday? (This was very much part of the "culture" when I was growing up.)

I invite you to WAIT (remember "What Am I Thinking?" in Chapter 4?). The yoga therapy practice I am talking about in this chapter is about relaxing the brainbody, known as "the yoga of sleep." During a Yoga Nidra session, you will be invited to lie on a yoga mat or sit in a chair and participate in a directed, imaginary journey around the body (with the eyes closed or covered), while taking a mindful elevator ride into deeper energetic brainwave states, accessing the subcortical brain, and landing in a state of deep rest. From this relaxed falling awake state of mind in Yoga Nidra, all that is holding you back in your life can be brought to the surface for the cortical brain to consider and release without comment. Don't let the name Yoga Nidra or the reference to "the yoga of sleep" fool you; this practice is more about learning how to train yourself to stop, relax, wake up, let go, and fall awake (Kabat-Zinn 2018; Moore 2019). Right now, your cortical brain may be saying, "Huh? You mean I don't have to strike a pose? Then how does it work?" If you are asking yourself this as you start to read this chapter, great! This means you are "falling awake!"

While yoga has a very long, rich tradition and history of healing and transformative practices across cultures, it often remains misunderstood and is viewed as a novel or alternative form of "exercise" in the United States (Gurda 2015). According to Swami Rama (1996), founder and spiritual head of the Himalayan Institute in Honesdale, Pennsylvania,

> [t]he majority of people view yoga only as a system of physical culture. Very few understand that the science behind yoga and the Yoga Nidra practice is complete in itself. When one is trained to teach Yoga Nidra, you learn the neuroscience and energetic shifts that systematically access the subcortical brain with body sensing, breath awareness, focusing the mind, and intentional practices. When one understands that a human being is not only a physical being but a breathing being and thinking being too, then the research does not limit itself to the body and breath only. Gaining control over the mind and its modifications, and the feelings and emotions, becomes more important than practicing a few postures or breathing exercises. (1996, pp.xvii–xix)

> *If the restraint of the mental modifications is achieved one has reached the goal of Yoga. The entire science of Yoga is based on this. (**The Yoga Sutras of Patanjali 1.2**)*

Yoga Nidra is a brainbody therapy

As presented earlier in this book, the recognition of the impact of past events on the mind, brain, and body acknowledges the limitations of cognitive processing in traditional talk therapy alone. When considering Yoga Nidra as a brainbody therapy for relaxing the nervous system to heal the impact of trauma and other life events, we may still need to shift and update our perspectives about how these (memories, stress, etc.) access, land, and become trapped inside of us. Recovery from the impact of events is neurological, somatic, and physiological. Yoga Nidra is considered a horizontal meditation (Dinsmore-Tuli 2014; Dinsmore-Tuli and Tuli 2022). During its practice, these are accessed and regulated through a gradual, energetic, systematic, therapeutic process. The brainbody responds the same way to stress, whether it is to a shooting, argument, bombing, war, divorce, violence, addiction, natural or man-made disaster, or chronic health issue. We know we can get stuck, keeping the accelerator pressed, leading to sympathetic dominance.

Living in a constant state of emergency (anxiety, panic, fear, pressure, or over-whelm, etc.) triggers the release of neurochemicals, such as cortisol, and engages the fight, flight, freeze, or faint response (that PVT/brain forest stuff again). This constant alarm fluctuation of the nervous system can create intense mental turmoil, tension, and sometimes pain in the body, which, when held over time, can become chronic reactive ways of experiencing the world. This prolonged hyperarousal state of mind can be very disruptive to daily life and exhausting for the physical body (causing elevated blood pressure, increased heart rate, muscle tension, inflammation, etc.), especially when there is no current cause for alarm to flee for safety, or chaos to dismantle. Constantly being "on guard" and in a state of hypervigilance is draining. This activated "felt sense" experience of being unable to calm down or self-regulate (impaired concentration and memory, difficulty sleeping) can present in us as a lack of motivation, and increased inability to find a sense of purpose—as no one and no where is "safe." Simultaneously, this can then engage the Committee or the default mode network (DMN) (known as maladaptive rumination—or need for drama—all referred to earlier), which become the "normal" way of existing and being in daily stressful events. When present-oriented awareness is "offline" or inaccessible, the switch to turn on the inner chat room of the mind (the Committee, Monkey Mind) "flipping our lid" (discussed in Chapter 1) is triggered. This heightened emotional state remains activated while the person responds to the memory, stress, or past trauma that was triggered as if it is happening in real time, as if it is happening *now* (remember the amygdala alarm center discussion—yes, back to the brain forest!).

The practice of Yoga Nidra helps the person develop body and breath awareness, according to Dr. Ray Long (2005, 2008), an orthopedic surgeon and founder of Bandha yoga, or "psychic sleep." He notes that Huberman's phrase "non-sleep deep rest" effectively describes Yoga Nidra. Through learning the basics of the musculoskeletal groups that become tight and tense in response to stress (Kami-noff and Matthews 2011), relaxing and visualizing these parts during Yoga Nidra's progressive relaxation can shift "thinking" by reorienting to the present moment. Throughout this book there has been an invitation to learn about and study brain-body basics in order to realize the temporary reactive state of the mind, body, and breath, which we can control. This is highly recommended because in order to deeply know ourselves, we must take the journey within our physical brainbody. Shifting the narrative about what is going on with intense feelings, memories, emo-tions, and physical pain can be difficult, especially when attached to "the story" that became "normal" ways of thinking, living, and being (Miller 2015; J. Miller 2023). To be aware of and observe these mental and physical states with detached awareness is difficult, and to release, let them go, or shift them, even more so (Forbes 2011).

Miller's (2010b) research and iRest program (2015) on the effectiveness of Yoga Nidra for overcoming trauma for veterans diagnosed with PTSD, along with van der Kolk's (2014) work, recognized that witness consciousness or mindful experience without reaction, using yoga skills like Yoga Nidra, can help clients regulate the brainbody (Cope 2006; Kabat-Zinn 1994). The application of these skills teaches clients focused attention and awareness of sensations in the body, creating the feeling of being mindfully present in time and space...not being in the past or future, just being right where you are in this moment. The skills and benefits developed in various yoga practices, including Yoga Nidra, has fueled research and endorsement for yoga as an integral part of trauma-informed psychotherapy and yoga therapy sessions (Gard *et al.* 2014). The impact of trauma or other events leaves a lasting imprint in the neurological, sensory, and hormonal systems, often leaving the client "afraid to be in their own skin," referring back to the "issues in the tissues" (Khalsa 2008; La Barre 2010; Leela 2022; Rosen 2014).

Yoga Nidra is considered by some as a longer, deeper form of meditation or "psychic sleep." Huberman coined the phrase "non-sleep deep rest" and Miller "iRest" to use with other populations (e.g., the military, schoolteachers, corporate CEOs) who may be turned off when they hear the word "yoga" (Miller 2023). The process of Yoga Nidra practice accesses deep states of consciousness that can ignite lasting change as a person moves through the different brainwave states that awaken their true nature. Yoga Nidra practice includes the following phases: establishing a comfortable secure position and space; setting an intention; focused awareness of physical sensation; guided relaxation around the body; use of breath; accessing energy layers (the five koshas); awareness of cognitions and imagery; and returning to the wakeful present moment. Desai (2017) describes using the tools of Yoga Nidra during these phases of the practice as mentally removing our "sunglasses" and beginning to see life through a different lens...hence having the experience falling awake.

The five brainwave states accessed during Yoga Nidra are:

- Beta (conscious mind, normal waking state): This is the awake alert state of mind (such as that engaged when reading this book or watching a movie), getting things done, very task-oriented.

- Gamma (optimal mental state): Although most frequently experienced when awake, this is the brainwave that organizes memory and long-term learning. Gamma can also be experience during REM sleep.

- Alpha (relaxed and calm brain state, physical relaxation): Considered the state of dreaming. Shifting from awake and crossing the bridge to being asleep. In Yoga Nidra, this is the state of noticing "thinking" without reacting or engaging, just letting go. It is in the alpha state that images, memories, and events come and go.

- Theta (deeply relaxed or meditative, deep-sleep brain state, comfortably numb while sober): Dream, imagery, sense of here but not here. The theta state is where Yoga Nidra is stilling the fluctuations of the mind referred to earlier.

- Delta (pure consciousness): This is the deep calm state of silence, the state of turiya, or the fourth state of consciousness, (the movement through three states of waking, dreaming, and deep sleep that occurs via the corresponding brainwaves to access turiya). In the language of yoga, turiya is the state of consciousness beyond waking, dreaming, and dreamless, deep sleep. In some Yoga Nidra practices, it is called the relaxed state of mind or landing at the bottom of the ocean. While more study is needed, the delta brainwave state accessed during Yoga Nidra preserves cognitive ability after trauma. It is speculated that Yoga Nidra could be an important tool to enhance recovery from traumatic brain injury because of the slow-wave delta brainwave state it induces (Desai 2017).

According to Sovik (2005), the systematic relaxation techniques used during the Yoga Nidra session is what he calls "the heart of the relaxation process." This involves mentally travelling around and through the body from one part to the next. He explains that, through this imaginary journey, Yoga Nidra teaches practitioners to learn how to know about and relax the body better, become aware of how to control the mind, and experience how the mind has control of the body. During the energetic, deep relaxation experience of Yoga Nidra (the journey through the five koshas and five brainwave states), participants often report the experience of hovering between a waking and sleeping state of attentive relaxation. Yoga Nidra often begins with an intention or focus for the practice and can also involve exploring the inner world through visual imagery, sensations, feelings, and possibilities for the future (Ryba 2022).

In the profound state of relaxation that can occur during the practice of Yoga Nidra, the laser-focused mind, along with the sequence of techniques and steps just mentioned, awakens and harnesses the extraordinary power and wisdom of the mindbody, inviting spontaneous healing through the ability to access the past and future (Tigunait 2019). There are enormous raw emotions and radical healing that can happen during Yoga Nidra. The physical position of lying down (which can feel vulnerable for some) and the relief of not having to talk while reaching the deep subcortical parts of the brain (you don't have to share or give the details of what you experience, like in EMDR or BSP) can be one of the "gems" experienced. Long says the theta brainwave states of Yoga Nidra engage the intuitive unconscious mind accessing deep-seated memories where healing occurs (Miller 2023). Although Yoga Nidra offers many benefits and treasures, it does require practice, and its repetition disciplines the mind towards stillness.

The psychology behind yoga and Yoga Nidra is breaking habitual patterns, such as refraining from reacting and responding to events with intense emotions or destructive numbing-out behaviors (Shivapremananda 1997). Yoga practice is about learning to occupy and stay in the brainbody—to be fully present, to sit, stand, balance, lie down, and relax with conscious awareness. Sometimes everything gets better when we unplug for a moment to let our brainbody reset and recalibrate.

My yoga story

I discovered yoga during the 1980s in New York City, when I was attending New York University, and became very curious about this yoga center called Jivamukti, created by Sharon Gannon and David Life (2002). Here I found out about the benefits of the yoga poses, the benefits of lifestyle-based daily self-care and spiritual practices (Gannon 2018), and the science of Ayurveda (Sivananda Yoga Vedanta Center 2018; see also Leela 2022; Lad 2009; Yarema, Rhoda, and Brannigan 2006). Yoga was considered very avant-garde and innovative at the time. Without Jivamukti and many internationally acclaimed teachers and public speakers, yoga would still be seen as an obscure practice for vegans who speak Sanskrit and do headstands. These teachers and speakers include: Seane Corn (2019), founder of the nonprofit Off the Mat Into the World® (OTM);[1] Amy Weintraub (2004, 2012, 2021), yoga therapist, author, and creator of LifeForce Yoga®; Durga Leela, founder of Yoga of Recovery (2022), yoga teacher, clinical ayurvedic specialist, and recovery coach; Nikki Meyers, founder of Y12SR, Yoga of 12-Step Recovery;[2] Lilias Folan (2005), author of Yoga Gets Better with Age; Peggy Cappy, creator of Yoga for the Rest of Us on PBS in 2007;[3] Angela Farmer, for over 40 years the teacher of "modern yoga" using a feminine non-lineage style; and Reggie Hubbard, creator of Active Peace Yoga in 2014,[4] bringing transformative practices like Yoga Nidra and sound bowl healing yoga retreats to men of color; and many others.

Yes, there is much for you to explore, learn, and obtain training or take a class in to experience the many healing practices that have their beginnings in yoga. Dr. John Douillard,[5] author of *Body, Mind, and Sport* (1994), was also a major influence in my introduction to yoga since there were not many studios around at the time his book published. It introduced me to sun salutations and followed the step-by-step instructions on how to teach them to myself. Then I discovered Beth Shaw's non-lineage YogaFit® (2009) yoga teacher training, which appealed to me because of its focus on exercise for the fitness industry. I completed my 500-hour training in 2009 and did not appreciate all the additional "gems" of yoga (like Yoga Nidra) beyond the physical poses until much later.

Much later, because of low back pain from running (literally) and preparing for the New York City marathon (several times) during the early 1990s, I went to an orthopedic doctor who told me I needed back surgery (of course he recommended surgery—that is the focus of his training). When I read Dr. John Sarno's book *Healing Back Pain* (1991), in which he does not suggest surgery for back pain, I decided to get a second opinion. The next doctor I saw told me I did not need surgery; he told me I needed to do yoga. I was in so much back pain from being a runner I could not fathom (and many people still react this way) how yoga can possibly be helpful (I

---

1   www.offthematintotheworld.org
2   www.y12sr.com/team
3   https://peggycappy.com
4   https://activepeaceyoga.com
5   https://lifespa.com

can't bend over, do a back bend, or stand on my head—I felt that then and people think this when they hear the word "yoga"). The only yoga studio around at the time was offering what is called Bikram Yoga. Bikram yoga, now referred to as "hot yoga," was created by Bikram Choudhury (1978), a yoga teacher from India. Classes consist of a fixed sequence of 26 postures[6] done at every class, practiced in a room heated to 105°F, intended to replicate the climate of India. The room is fitted with carpets and the walls are covered in mirrors. Not able to move or bend because I was in so much back pain, I just sat in the back of the room on the floor, watched the others, and sweated. One day, when I attempted to do one of the stretches from a kneeling position, my lower back literally "popped" back into place. It felt like a miracle—without surgery—and this miracle moment hooked me into researching the healing potential of yoga, leading me to learn more about other schools of yoga and eventually become a yoga teacher and a certified yoga therapist. I learned about the healing practice of Yoga Nidra during the completion of my yoga teacher training in India.

While learning about the benefits of integrating yoga practices into the psychotherapy session, I met Amy Weintraub (2004, 2012), author and yoga leader and creator of LifeForce Yoga® training for healthcare professionals. Graduating from her program, I assisted Amy in her programs, teaching health professionals and co-trained with her to teach mental health and addiction professionals the self-care practices of yoga involved in self-regulation. She also was instrumental to me in learning the benefits of an Ayurvedic lifestyle and Yoga Nidra when she helped me go to India (she and Sue Tebb organized a fundraiser for me) to detox from the impact of chemotherapy and radiation and learn about Yoga Nidra. Durga Leela, author of *Yoga of Recovery: Integrating Yoga and Ayurveda with Modern Recovery Tools for Addiction* and creator of the 12 Steps, is also one of my teachers. She conducts yearly month-long retreats focusing on this in South India.[7]

Yoga Nidra snapshot

Yoga Nidra is composed of systematic instructions that guide you imaginally inside the body into gradually deeper states of muscle relaxation and present-state awareness. It can be practiced in 5-, 10-, or 20-minute sessions, although a full Yoga Nidra experience is usually 30–45 minutes. Depending on the group and location for Yoga Nidra, clients may engage in some gentle stretching or tense and release cues to relax any muscle tension. After setting the stage for the practice with a focused sankalpa or intention (see Appendix C), or identifying what stress, worry, or craving they want to let go of during the practice, clients are cued to land on their back (or to sit on a chair) and observe the whole body resting while they slow down their breathing. Clients are invited to choose from a mental imagery offered or to use one of their

---

6   https://en.wikipedia.org/wiki/Postures_of_Bikram_Yoga
7   https://yogaofrecovery.com/calendar

own, notice sensations, memories, and emotions present to release, and then finally rest in the experience of silence. This is when the release of intense feelings and emotions can happen organically and naturally, without effort, or the realization that this is actually happening (the cortical brain is offline here).

The experience of Yoga Nidra practice begins a fascinating journey of discovery by going within. As it becomes more popular, it aims to revise our cultural appreciation of sleep and reverse our neglect of it (Walker, 2017). Yoga Nidra asks you to lie down and wake up—no movement, talking, or thinking required! You can do Yoga Nidra with eyes open or closed in a chair or lying on your side, back, or stomach. Doing this practice regularly, you should find that instead of falling asleep, it is possible to train yourself to fall awake (Kabat-Zinn 2018).

Some yoga lineages specifically require the eyes to be open or closed (in which case, eye coverings can be helpful). However, specific setups, props used, and the type of Yoga Nidra session provided depends on the circumstances—mainly, who is leading the practice, where Yoga Nidra is being offered, and the population/clients who are doing it (a group class or one-to-one).

The origins of Yoga Nidra

Yoga Nidra was first written about in a yoga text called the *Upanishads*, which is about self-realization, and is estimated to have been written about 700 BCE, making it more than 2000 years old—almost 1000 years before the birth of Jesus! With origins in an oral tradition that likely dates even further back in time, it was considered a manifestation of the power of the Goddess Devi.

In more modern times, Sigmund Freud, considered "the father of psychiatry," was an unconscious recliner. It is thought that around 1890, a grateful "cured" female patient gifted Freud a Victorian daybed, leading him to introduce the couch into his practice, which then became the staple furniture of the psychotherapy session. Freud even brought the famed couch with him when he came to the United States in 1909! While not a yoga practice, psychoanalysis certainly holds similarities with Yoga Nidra in its focus on relaxation and allowing the mind to turn its attention to what arises from within. In 1891, author Annie Payson-Call wrote a book entitled *Power Through Repose* in which she described the state of "Nidra" as a state of pure awareness—proprioceptive relaxation. Payson-Call was concerned with the fast pace of modern life and the effects on mental health. In the focus of her movement trainings, she pioneered education on the role of language, body awareness, imagination, and sensory knowledge in releasing muscle tension.

Most recently, the arrival of spiritual teachers from the East helped to introduce and spread the knowledge and practices of Yoga Nidra. Swami Satyananda Saraswati (1976) is considered the first teacher to have popularized and written about Yoga Nidra meditation in its current form in a book known as the "Blue Book," offered by the Bihar school of yoga in India. Adapted from tantric texts, he formulated the basis of this technique while serving as a disciple of his guru, the great yoga master Swami

Sivananda, in Rishikesh, India, during the 1940s and early 1950s. Swami Satyananda describes how, as a young student, he fell asleep while a nearby group of people chanted mantras—many of which he had not heard before. Even though he was deeply asleep during the chanting, when he awoke and heard these mantras again, he seemed to know them. A yogi explained to Swami Satyananda that his *subtle body* had heard the mantras. The characteristic feature of Yoga Nidra meditation is the systematic rotation of consciousness in the body, which originated from the tantric process of nyasa (meaning to place or to take the mind to a point).

In 1970, Swami Rama (1996) came to the United States and formed the Himalayan Institute in Honesdale, Pennsylvania, where his student and successor Dr. Pandit Rajmani Tigunait (2019) now serves as the spiritual head. Swami Kripalu came to the United States in 1977 for four years at the invitation of his student, Amrit Desai, who founded the first Kripalu Center in Pennsylvania with his wife and brother in 1972, and later a Kripalu ashram in Massachusetts. This inspired many people to start practicing yoga. In 1994 Amrit Desai left the Kripalu Ashram and went on to create the Integrative Amrit Method (I AM Method) of Yoga at the Amrit Institute in Florida. Shortly after, he founded the I AM Method of Yoga Nidra, which his daughter and successor, Dr. Kamini Desai (2017), built on to create the method we know today. Desai now teaches the method worldwide, as do other senior teachers, including John Vosler, a respected instructor and retreat leader in the field.

Perhaps no one has done more to make Yoga Nidra known in the West than Dr. Richard Miller, who created iRest, which integrates the practice with psychology for the treatment for PTSD (2015). His work has included studies of iRest with the military and "has been approved as a Complementary and Alternative Medicine warranting continuing research for use in the treatment of PTSD. In addition, the US Army Surgeon General has listed Yoga Nidra as a Tier 1 approach for addressing pain management in military care" (Miller 2015, p.2).

Many others have significantly contributed to the growth of knowledge about and use of Yoga Nidra, including Dr. Herbert Benson (1975), who created and wrote the book *The Relaxation Response* at Harvard after studying the meditation practices of Tibetan monks in the Himalayas. In 1977, Rod Stryker wrote *The Four Desires* and took up residency at the Himalayan Institute, where he created his version of Nidra practices, as did Rolf Sovik, who developed the 61 points and other Nidra practices. In 1979, Jon Kabat-Zinn launched the famed mindfulness-based stress reduction (MBSR) program at the University of Massachusetts Medical Center, where his work has been studied ever since, and serves to establish a clear scientific connection between modern practices that emerged from Eastern knowledge and traditions and their use in contemporary healthcare.

In 2004, Amy Weintraub published *Yoga for Depression* and founded the Life-Force Yoga® training institute, and created CDs for mental health professionals to bring Yoga Nidra and other yoga practices into the therapy session. (I am a trained instructor in LifeForce Yoga®.)

What happens during a Yoga Nidra session?

Just like the other brain therapies you have been reading about, Yoga Nidra bypasses the "upstairs" thinking brain and goes deep into the autonomic nervous system—the home of the sympathetic and parasympathetic nervous systems. The practice of Yoga Nidra quiets the inner noise of the thinking mind (the Committee, Monkey Mind) to make it easier to access your true nature (Desai 2017). A sankalpa or intention for the practice provides a *focus* for the Nidra session, and can be very valuable in the process of self-inquiry, learning, and self-healing (see Appendix C for sample sankalpas or intentions).

This focus, or mental statement of intention, during Yoga Nidra is followed by an energetic progressive relaxation of the marma points and major muscle groups around the body, while relaxing the breath, using imagery, and resting in silence (Parker, Bharati, and Fernandez 2013). This quieting of the mind provides the brain-body the opportunity to become comfortable with chaos and order, grief, and joy, being present or somewhere else—like being awake and asleep at the same time (Dinsmore-Tuli and Tuli 2022).

As you and/or your clients experience and practice Yoga Nidra regularly, you will come to see how beliefs, culture, and conditioning can fuel anxiety, panic, fear, guilt, shame, and other reactive physical and mental patterns that create suffering. During Yoga Nidra, these can be brought to the surface and released. This is done by guiding you/your client into deep relaxation and moving through various brainwave states (non-REM sleep) that the ancient yogis refer to as states of consciousness. Depending on the capacity and possibility of the practitioner to be still and relax, deep relaxation, pleasant experiences, past experiences, even the experience of levitation can occur (Saraswati 1976).

According to Desai:

> What is Yoga Nidra? It is like floating...floating is not something you do, it is something that is happening in the absence of doing. It is an experience of being held, being carried. But it can only happen when you stop struggling to keep upright. When you stop doing, floating happens. Stop efforting and sleep happens. When you let go of doing anything, everything gets done. This concept is so foreign to the Western mind, we can hardly fathom it. (2017, p.xi)

There is a reason stress is at epidemic levels in the West, and Desai believes this is why:

> We don't know how to stop. Our waking hours have taken over our sleeping hours. Even our sleep and rest is in the service of doing more rather than being more. We don't sleep to be rested, to revitalize, and nourish ourselves. We sleep so we can get up and do more the next day. We haven't mastered the art of non-doing with the art of doing. We haven't learned how to relax in action. This is another way to describe Yoga Nidra. (2017, p.xi)

Yoga Nidra, as well as The FUN® Program and the brain therapies shared in this book, bring into awareness all that is possible in your life. They gently clear intense emotions, blocking beliefs and stories that may be holding you back in your life, and help you transform them. The Yoga Nidra session is not only about being present in the body and mind, but also about allowing yourself to relax and lie or sit still, nothing required of you other than to remain fully awake. Research on Yoga Nidra shows that a 45-minute profound practice of relaxation (while remaining awake and alert throughout) is the equivalent of three hours of sleep! (See also Appendix D.)

When we are no longer lured by or attached to thinking and able to silence the mind, falling awake begins. Our thoughts and actions are revealed while we remain calm and in the present. Before 1960, Yoga Nidra was not widely known in the West (LeWine 2024). However, our understanding of how high levels of stress impact our mental and physical heath is not new: "Millions of patients all over the world who suffer from psychosomatic diseases can be helped through right diet, juices, relaxation, breathing, and meditation. Preventative and alternative medicine should not be ignored" (Rama 1978, p.348). Some instruct that the breathing should be deep, slow, smooth, silent, and continuous, but there are many ways to calm the breath down. The way we experience suffering is how it shows up in the mind, the body, and how we breathe.

> Marines will not respond to "fairy trauma yoga therapies." Marines are a unique closed tribe... General yoga for Veterans will not work... I stay away from the VA [Veterans' Association]. (Marine)

> We won't go to yoga even if offered by one of us [a cop]. To talk about or do some "trauma informed yoga" is breaking the code...we are supposed to know what to do to take care of ourselves. (Police officer)

Let's help the people who have served to protect our country (here in the United States and abroad) receive the gifts of brainbody exercises we can all do (us mental health people are doing our service too) to heal and stay on track:

> Breathe out through the mouth slowly and say to yourself: "Unshakable confidence and trust breathes through me now. Breathe in slowly: Everything I need exists within me. I have everything I need to manage my life." Repeat and say this to yourself three times (this is adapted from Amy Weintraub, LifeForce Yoga® training).

The healing aspects of yoga

Yoga practitioners use breathwork, a focus on sensation, and physical poses to connect the breath, body, and mind and to turn the attention inward. You can incorporate elements of yoga into your clinical work to help your clients finally break free from the immobilizing grip of emotions. Gard *et al.* (2014), in their comprehensive overview of research on yoga and its benefits on psychological health, provide evidence that shows yoga affecting self-regulatory pathways, integrating concepts from behavior therapy and cognitive neuroscience, with emerging yoga and meditation research. Their review of the literature—including the works and contributions of yoga leaders mentioned earlier in this chapter—suggest that yoga, specifically Yoga Nidra, can improve symptoms of depression, anxiety, stress, and PTSD, as well as promote well-being, including life satisfaction, inspire motivation and creativity, and overall happiness. There is no overall framework other than that by doing the practice we strengthen the skills of self- regulation. And according to Weintraub (2012), every aspect of yoga can be done in a variety of settings and ways: no yoga mat required.

How does Yoga Nidra embrace the neural network in healing? And what if you are saying to yourself "I'm not a yoga teacher, so how can I use it with my clients?" As your neural networks light up and get challenged in this section, you'll discover the neuroscience behind Yoga Nidra and how it can be an effective integrative practice for relief from trauma and other stress-related problems. Practical daily self-soothing exercises and applications will be offered that you can easily start using immediately in your practice. Long-term studies reveal that an ongoing yoga practice of some kind helps support and maintain these benefits.

Try Yoga Nidra yourself

You will find a full Yoga Nidra session in Appendix D, which was designed by Kamini Desai and myself specifically for this book, with the emphasis on the brainbody and healing. It can be helpful to record the script in advance to allow you to simply relax and follow the guiding prompts. When you are ready to begin, choose a comfortable, private place to lie down or sit, where you will not be interrupted for about 45 minutes. Also, have a blanket to hand as your body temperature will drop. Some people like to use an eye covering to support them in going within.

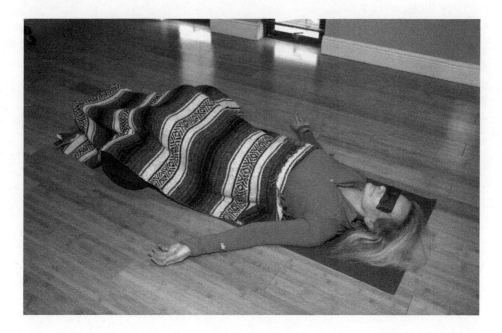

The first time, like beginning any new type of therapy or exercise, you or your client might be challenged by the Inner Critic, Skeptic, or other members of the Committee avoiding or not sure of the benefit of trying something new. The cortical brain may get involved "trying to figure out" alternatives to lying on the floor (chair, use of props, lying on one's side) and/or face the fact that the practice involves no talking or movement—just "lying down," fully awake for 40–45 minutes. This can be due to the belief of our fast-paced busy culture that doing "nothing" is a waste of time. Trust me, it's ultimately better than the nonstop chatter of the mind. And having the script as a guide helps to mitigate the "nothing," providing "something" to focus on.

I often use a shorter Yoga Nidra practice with my groups as a centering exercise. Its formal name is Vishoka Meditation (Aharana Pranayama), and it is taught at the Himalayan Institute. I have adapted it for use in any setting outside of a yoga center.

MY ADAPTED VISHOKA MEDITATION YOGA NIDRA SCRIPT

Sit in a comfortable seat with your head and neck aligned with a straight spine (if possible). Withdraw the mind from all distractions and just land here, right now, in this moment. You have chosen this time to take care of you. Notice your mind and body and the space it occupies as you settle in.

Take 5–7 long, smooth, relaxed breaths. Allow the breath to slow down and invite the mind to feel the gentle, slow, continuous quality of the flow of your breathing.

Now we begin an imaginary journey around the body with the eyes closed (or softened gaze). As we travel around the body, have your gentle focus on each location. You are only aware of the feeling of the breath at each location. At each location take one effortless inhale and exhale.

Let's begin: Bring your attention to the center of your forehead and allow your awareness to rest here. Remain relaxed and do not put any pressure on your eyes. Take 3 relaxed breaths here.

Now we begin the imaginary journey around the body. Take 1 relaxed inhale and exhale at each of these points:

- Center, between the eyebrows
- Eyes
- Nostrils
- Throat
- Both shoulders
- Both upper arms
- Both elbows
- Both wrists
- Both palms

Bring your attention to the fingertips and take 2 complete breaths. Next, take 1 complete breath at the:

- Palms
- Wrists
- Elbows
- Upper arms
- Shoulders

- Throat
- Heart
- Bottom of the sternum
- Navel center
- Pelvis

Take 2 complete breaths at the perineum. Then take 1 complete breath at the:

- Pelvis
- Navel center
- Bottom of the sternum
- Heart

- Throat
- Nostrils
- Eyes
- Eyebrow center

Bring your attention to the center of the forehead and take 3–5 breaths.

Finally, release all effort and allow your awareness to be held effortlessly by the space at the center of the forehead. Enjoy the stillness and vibrancy of this space.

When you are ready, gently deepen your breathing and land back in your body, breathe out through your mouth slowly, and open your eyes.

There are many online resources for you to experience Yoga Nidra, including video and audio recordings as well as apps (including the I AM Yoga Nidra app). There are short practices and long practices, Yoga Nidra for sleep, Yoga Nidra for relaxation, etc.—try one and find what works best for you! You can also ask at the yoga studio(s) near you whether they offer Yoga Nidra sessions.

Bringing somatics into the therapy office

Somatic therapy is having a conversation about sensations and where we feel these in our body. We can start with the five senses: smell, taste, sight, sound, touch. Describing what is happening when the body is shaking, the voice quivering, the head pounding, the back aching, the mind racing with words, breath, and movement using the five senses is somatic therapy. The sensations in the body alert us to the present moment.

How do we use the self-soothing, often somatically based, exercises available today to calm the body, release tension, erase cravings, and restore mindbody balance in the office? By trying them out, experimenting, using them ourselves, and sharing them with clients. It is easy because these tools are portable. We can take them and use them anywhere, any time. These self-soothing tools are always around, and so is the inner addict (the one having cravings and thinking about drinking/drug use) and the outer addict (gambling, gaming, smoking, over-eating, television and social media compulsion). The Committee (Monkey Mind) shows up as self-hatred and the behavioral symptoms show up as cravings, rage, and eventual substance misuse.

Change happens when there is a willingness to connect with your own wisdom and confidence instead of going for that short-term symptom relief.

What can be the root problem? Self-absorption and reactive feelings, aka ego clinging: stay at the party, or remain in the relationship because of fear of being talked about, being alone, or other "stories" about "what if" (the Committee is in charge). Trying to maintain what we think is security, happiness, comfort—the three zones of safety—can create suffering. When we are not in present time (paying attention to DEAD (the Committee) or not feeling safe, secure or at ease, we have the compulsion to be distracted and engage in unhealthy, immediate, comfort-seeking behaviors. This is the background hum of restlessness, being triggered to use a substance, or other sympathetic nervous activation. Doing "nothing" or mindful self-care during these instances can be hard to engage in as the amygdala and cortical brain are always seeking something to hold on to (yes, back to the brain forest).

For example, when we have a scratch, an itch, a discomfort...we scratch it and get temporary relief. What if the doctor/teacher gives the "prescription" to stay with the scratch or sensation instead of trying to escape the bad feeling, worry, craving? When you stop scratching or using and apply the teaching or the work, healing happens. However, please be patient if you are new to these concepts. Learning them and integrating what works for you and your healing takes time.

Here are some examples to cue to somatic sensation in the body:

- Touch: placing the hand on the belly, shoulder, heart, or clasping the hands, giving yourself a hug, or splashing water on the face.

- Sound: sounds coming from a distance, music (a song you are thinking about), the sound of water, the sound of birds.

- Smell: lavender, the air, flowers, mint, favorite food, the smell of a pet.

- Taste: lemon, cool water, mint, spicy, sweet.

- Sight: beach, mountain, concert, river, stream, mountain.

Yoga Nidra, like the other brain therapies, is more curious about our attention to intention. Which brings us back to F in The FUN® Program...what is our focus for the practice or session?

The breath is another simple, wonderful tool for connecting to the present moment of the body. Pranayama (conscious breathing) is referred to throughout the practice of Yoga Nidra. Calm inhalations into the nostrils and longer exhales out through the mouth are commonly suggested. Left nostril breathing calms, right nostril energizes, breath of joy combines movement, breath, and sound. Bellows breath, bee's breath. When the mind wanders, come back to the breath.

Now for a word about props. While yoga studios may be full of them, as therapists, we can invest in a few small items or use what we have:

- A thick, sticky yoga mat with a folded blanket placed over it to make it more comfortable.

- A wall for those seated on a chair. Back the chair up against the wall and lay the head back on it for support (to prevent the head dropping forward).

- A cushion/pillow/bolsters to support the body behind the knees.

- Eye covers/pillows are very nice (a washcloth works well).

- A blanket to cover up (the body often cools down during the practice). Blankets can also be used to provide support for the knees, ankles, or around the head to support the neck.

You can expand on somatic awareness exercises by introducing physical exercises, stretches, and movement. Movement of any kind is now seen as essential medicine. These are not required or necessary to gain the benefits of a Yoga Nidra session, but they can help prepare for lying down and relaxing. They are also wonderful for people—yourself or your clients—who naturally desire more physicality or to "shake things up" to bypass the thinking mind or to shift one's mood. Additionally, they can help keep the joints and muscle tissues flexible, freshen the skin, and keep the internal organs functioning optimally.

Some suggestions for movement or stretching before lying down include (all are optional):

- Standing pose

- Marching in place with arm swings

- Neck stretches (tilting the head gently from side to side)

- Shoulder shrugs towards the ears, relaxing them back down away from the ears

- Body shaking all over

- Gentle twists with arm swings or arm raises

- Hands over head and lift onto toes

- Toe/hand joints (make fists).

Then, once on the ground or seated in a chair:

- Foot flexion

- Ankle rotation

- Leg raises/double-leg vibration/forward bend

- Cat/cow (back flexions)

- Leg extensions

- Bridge

- Happy baby.

Trauma-informed yoga

According to Spence (2021) and to the Substance Abuse and Mental Health Services Administration (SAMHSA 2023), "There is a six-step approach to being trauma-informed: 1) safety, 2) trustworthiness and transparency, 3) peer support, 4) collaboration and mutuality, 5) empowerment and choice, and 6) cultural, historical, and gender issues." These steps are intentionally broad and general because being trauma-informed is not about a checklist (script) or an approach *per se*. Rather, being trauma-informed "requires constant attention, caring awareness, sensitivity, and possible cultural change" at multiple levels and constant checking for quality improvement (CDC 2020). This is true whether you work in private practice, a hospital, government-run agency, or not-for-profit organization.

Trauma-sensitive/informed yoga instruction incorporates a combination of meditation, mindfulness, mental imagery, breathing exercises, and physical postures (Weintraub 2012), all of which are modified depending on the population and clinical setting. Yoga is an integrative modality and is thought of as part of a clinical team or program—not necessarily as a stand-alone treatment method. The Trauma Research Foundation, under the leadership of Bessel van der Kolk, has set up the following five parameters or guidelines for trauma-informed yoga:

1. Environment: The rooms are free from distractions, clients are given the choice of posture (sit, stand, lie down), and do not have their backs to doors or exits.

2. Exercises and instructions are slow and carefully guided; options are provided to adjust or modify.

3. Teachers/instructors are trained within their scope of practice and qualified to teach the trauma-informed/sensitive yoga components.

4. Language is calm, caring, comforting, inclusive, and supportive (tone of voice should also be soft, and loud enough so all can hear you). The use of Sanskrit, the language of yoga, and making reference to deities is not recommended, unless this is discussed prior to the session (clients tell you or ask questions about faith and religious practices or preferences).

STUCK AND DEPRESSED

I had a client who was 72 and came to therapy at my office after her wife of many years died from a long struggle with cancer. She was not motivated to do anything and reported feeling "stuck." Here is what she reported to me after doing EMDR and Yoga Nidra back-to-back (on Zoom):

> I think that there might be something to an EMDR and Yoga Nidra combo. We did EMDR Tuesday and Yoga Nidra last night. The next day, I was doing stuff all afternoon: laundry, straightening things up, taking care of business stuff that's been "hanging." The same thing happened the last time I did EMDR and Yoga Nidra on the same day. The two together seem to work for me.

RESIDENTIAL ADDICTION TREATMENT

Here are the results of some data collected from doing Yoga Nidra at a residential addiction treatment center. The age range of men and women who attended the one-hour class (designated as a "mindful group exercise") was 18 to 67, and participants came from all over the United States. Their "drugs of choice" included meth, alcohol, clonidine, benzos, opiates, heroin, hydrocodone, and pot.

Like people at my psychotherapy office, as soon as I said, "Welcome to Yoga Nidra," the hyperfocus was on the word "yoga," implying to them a practice of doing head stands or putting the body into awkward positions. The immediate response was, "I can't do yoga," followed by a litany of pains and problems about getting on the floor on a yoga mat.

The participants filled out a questionnaire before and after the class to reveal what was upsetting them at first and what they found helpful when the class was over. After briefly introducing myself, we went right into the exercise. It was their choice whether to remain seated in a chair or lie on the floor on a yoga mat, and I explained that there would be no movement, talking, or sharing in the class. Consent to participate was included.

Here are some of the negative beliefs they shared about what contributed to their substance abuse/addiction (in addition to other situational factors or past traumas that were driving their use):

- Losing a job

- A controlling spouse

- Anxiety

- Past regrets

- Family chaos

- Being a bad parent

- People pleasing.

They also shared statements like: "I can't handle things," "I am a mess, something is wrong with me," "I am defective," "I am a failure," "I am a disappointment," "I am weak and not in control," and "Everything is my fault."

After the Yoga Nidra session, these were some of the important insights the participants shared having gained from the practice:

I can accept the true nature of myself... I am a good person.

Things I have done in the past are not important now. I can start over.

I know I have choices now. I am not defective or a total loss.

I am now in control. I am good enough.

I now have tools to accomplish my dreams.

It is possible to be happy and content—without alcohol or drugs.

I can fully relax, even without my contacts in!

My brain is very powerful—control of everything starts with relaxation.

Ethics and caution

While introductory work with somatic awareness or body movement can be done by anyone, only those with training and certification should be using EMDR, Brainspotting, or Yoga Nidra in their practice. Always begin by trying things out and doing the work on yourself first. As a healthcare practitioner or seeker of self-care, always think about your level of training, understanding, and scope of practice when utilizing any practice. When you are unsure, lack information, or face challenges, always seek out consultation with someone who knows more or has experience.

Because of the profound discoveries, revelations, and/or healing shifts that can occur when using these practices, every time you plan to use them, engage in some self-inquiry. Ask yourself: What is my motive? Is it to heal myself or to help others? Do I feel competent and understand why I am using this technique/practice? Before I learned about these, what was I doing for myself and using with my clients? This quick self-assessment will help you think about why and what you are doing. And if the answer is "I don't know" or "I am not sure," either seek out more training or obtain consultation from a master teacher or trainer.

When we are less stressed, taking time to rest, we become healthier and more prone to being at peace (Lusk 2021). The practice of Yoga Nidra can help us remain calm, no matter what is going on in our life, so our thinking brain can consider new options and be at peace. And it is possible to retrain our brain and experience change from the inside that we didn't even know was possible.

CHAPTER 5: VOCABULARY/FOLLOW-UP CONCEPTS

Here are some words and topics about Yoga Nidra for your further study and reference:

- Chakra
- Deity
- Dosha
- Energy/prana
- I AM Yoga Nidra (also an app for your phone)
- Ida
- iRest
- Karma
- Koshas
- Lineage
- Mental imagery/visualization
- Mindfulness
- Monkey Mind
- Namaste
- Opposite feelings and sensations
- Pingala
- Pratyahara
- Samskaras
- Sankalpa (intention)
- Sanskrit
- Savasana (corpse pose)
- Self-inquiry
- Sound bath
- Source
- Turiya

CHAPTER 6

The Power of Beliefs—How Our Stories Become Real!

As you continue falling awake, I hope that you are seeing how the beliefs and "stories" we hold in our mind about ourselves and our lives have the potential to have a lot of power over us—often revisiting us in the form of the Committee and Monkey Mind chatter. These often negative, destructive, critical beliefs and stories can be crippling and quite controlling. These habitual ways of thinking can make it quite challenging to consider or work toward embracing empowering and helpful ways of viewing situations. When talking—aloud to ourselves or to others—our thoughts and the words we use can have a strong impact on the well-being of the nervous system of the brain forest and the body. When we say, "I'm worried sick," or "My heart is broken," or "You're suffocating me," or "I'd rather be dead," unless we are awake and paying attention, we are firing off unwitting messages that we can ill afford to keep fertilizing. Unhelpful or limiting beliefs block the limitless ways we can see ourselves and what is possible for our present and future life. These unhelpful beliefs often grew up with us (becoming the Committee, Monkey Mind), and we are not only creating them but also becoming them (remember, they are our friends—protectors, defense, sympathetic, dorsal vagal systems). This is how the power of falling awake is possible and important.

Negative inner dialogue, self-inflicted judgment, or limiting, unhelpful beliefs (I don't like to refer to them as negative beliefs), particularly when issued as statements of "fact" by yourself or an "authority" such as your doctor, parents, teachers, employer, coach, or therapist, can impact you throughout your lifetime. Your behavior, thoughts, words, and the way you express your suffering is the "normal" that was created based on what was going on for you at that time in your life. How could you possibly know there is another way to look at or believe about situations that have occurred unless you looked at the ACE Questionnaire (ACE-Q), the Impact of Events Scale (IES) (Brown *et al.* 2015), or the Blocking Beliefs Questionnaire (BBQ) (Knipe 1998)? The healing journey with brain therapies can help you "see the big picture."

Falling and staying awake occurs with some kind of commitment to daily self-care (we all know what happens when we don't brush our teeth, or bathe—yuck). Ritualized, compulsive comfort-seeking (eating, drinking alcohol, smoking/vaping, constant yelling) are signals to take notice and consider what we are trying to feel or avoid. Using brain therapies can help to reveal and understand what happened, and how these patterns of coping were developed. Using our mental remote control to move from the "History" channel to the "Discovery" network may take time as we carefully explore our beliefs and behavior.

This is where we revisit the question from Chapter 1: Do your beliefs create your experiences, or do your experiences create your beliefs? Our current thoughts, stories, and beliefs do not appear randomly out of "the blue," but arise from the stories and underlying beliefs we have been carrying around mindlessly for a long time. Something about this fixation, attachment, or hard wiring usually comes from something that happened to us (Mintie and Staples 2018).

Your Committee (yes, the inner chat room or Monkey Mind you created) can have a field day with your limiting beliefs and thoughts. It thrills them to create worst-case scenarios and comparisons that reduce you to the size of a bug (think of being stuck in a tent with a fly). When blocking beliefs have taken up residence in your head, the Committee won't hesitate to use them to suit its own best interests, which you can be certain do not coincide with what is in your best interests.

Blocking beliefs

Sometimes a client's (or our) blocking belief(s) about an illness, diagnosis, addiction, trauma, abuse, grief, failed relationship, etc. will be right out there and apparent to both client and therapist, and it can be useful to ask some version of this question, "Even though you believe right now there is no way out from this, would it be all right with you to explore how you can?"

Sometimes a blocking belief is not always so obvious, or can be sneaky, and so with clients who seem stuck for "no apparent reason," I have found it useful to ask them to fill out or look over the BBQ (Knipe 1998, 2018). The client can rate what is referred to as the Validity of Cognition (the VoC, as used in EMDR) for each statement (how much they believe it to be true, 1 being "not all" to 7 "totally true"), or they may discover which blocking belief they are attached to by just glancing at the questionnaire. Once the blocking beliefs are identified, there are many options. Borrowing from an EMDR, Brainspotting, or Yoga Nidra setup, the therapist can ask, "When you think about this issue or what happened, what would you prefer to think about yourself instead?" Or, if the preferred belief does not seem possible at this moment, the client can pick one that seems the most possible right now and the therapist can "install" this preferred belief with EMDR, Brainspotting eye position, or a sankalpa or intention for Yoga Nidra that is moving towards this preferred belief, despite the presence of the blocking belief. Surprisingly, this sometimes gets past the block and makes the preferred belief possible.

A client was working on a childhood sexual trauma committed by a family member and was blocked in resolving her anger by the belief (her activation around this has a Subjective Units of Distress Scale (SUDS) rating of 6). She identified the blocking belief as, "This is a problem that can only be resolved by them" (i.e., making up for or apologizing for their neglect, which, in this case, was not likely). I asked her to try saying out loud to herself, while I used bilateral stimulation (slow eye movements used in EMDR), the following statement: "I am doing the best I can, given the circumstances I was in. I am free now." The repetition of this statement, out loud, is typically helpful for the self-acceptance idea to begin to take hold, especially if the perpetrator has died (confronting or holding them accountable is not possible *now*). The client was then able to go back to being more considerate of *herself as a survivor* from a painful situation, which is now a painful memory.

The basic idea is to ask the client to repeat, with eye movements, Brainspotting, eye position, tapping, or with a sankalpa or intention: "I accept [I love, I am loyal to, I can forgive] myself even though [insert blocking belief]." You can then go back to the issue to see if unblocked processing can resume.

QUESTIONNAIRE FOR ASSESSING BLOCKING BELIEFS

Go through the Blocking Belief Questionnaire together with the client and ask them to please give a number from 1 (feels completely untrue) to 7 (feels completely true) for each statement and go from there.

- [ ] I'm embarrassed that I have this problem.
- [ ] I will never get over this problem.
- [ ] I'm not sure I want to get over this problem.
- [ ] If I solve this problem, I will feel deprived.
- [ ] I don't have the strength or the willpower to solve this problem.
- [ ] If I really talk about this problem, something bad will happen.
- [ ] This is a problem that can only be solved by someone else.
- [ ] If I ever solve this problem, I will lose a part of who I really am.
- [ ] I don't want to think about this problem anymore.
- [ ] I should solve this problem, but I don't always do what I should.
- [ ] I like people who have this problem better than people who don't.
- [ ] It could be dangerous for me to get over this problem.
- [ ] When I try to think about this problem, I can't keep my mind on it.

- [ ] I say I want to solve this problem, but I never do.

- [ ] It could be bad for someone else for me to get over this problem.

- [ ] If I get over this problem, I can never go back to having it again.

- [ ] I don't deserve to get over this problem.

- [ ] This problem is bigger than I am.

- [ ] If I got over this problem, it would go against my values.

- [ ] Someone in my life hates this problem.

- [ ] There are some good things about having this problem.

- [ ] I don't have a problem.

- [ ] I've had this problem so long; I could never completely solve it.

- [ ] I have to wait to solve this problem.

- [ ] If I solve this problem, I could lose a lot.

- [ ] If I solve this problem, it will be mainly for someone else.

The BBQ can be very useful for addressing negative thoughts or strong beliefs held about a past traumatic event or situation. For more information about how to use this and other EMDR-related tools for complex PTSD and dissociation, check out Knipe's work (1998).

Blocking beliefs and the Committee

You may remember meeting the Committee from Chapter 2 (and you can find detailed information in Appendix B). Both the Committee and our Monkey Mind are involved with our blocking beliefs—creating them and enforcing them. When we begin the work of dismantling our blocking beliefs and creating boundaries with certain members of the Committee (you may have more tendency to jump up and down and scream), we gain more confidence about falling awake. Let's look at some members of the Committee who try to keep their power:

- The Storyteller comments on the future or the past and present.

- The Namer labels people, events, and diseases.

- The Shamer instills embarrassment, guilt, and fault.

- The Blamer says that you and others are at fault for the events and circumstances of your life.

- The Comparer elevates or devalues your worth depending on others.

- The Concluder says, "if this, then" jumps to habitual disasters for "stories."

- The Judge (also the Know It All) determines what is right from wrong, good from bad, normal from abnormal.

- The Social Arbitrator decides the acceptability and appropriateness of *everything*.

- The Victimizer makes you the injured party, either by your own hand or someone else's.

- The Skeptic makes you doubt even your own experience.

- The Inner Critic always questions everything you do (and often hangs out with the Skeptic).

The Committee and the blocking beliefs in the BBQ manipulate us with their constant demands for attention and power, and being aware of them can challenge the Monkey Mind. Just because these beliefs and their stories take place all in our own mind does not reduce their impact or mean they are not real. Sometimes the intensity of these "stories"—or what is revealed during the belief inventory or during a brain therapy session—may be one of the most profound revelations a person can encounter. Through the lens of the FUN® approach, the attunement that takes place between the therapist and client to *Focus* on and *Undo* these beliefs creates space for freedom. This frustrates the Committee, the Monkey Mind, and the default mode network (DMN), which all count on your beliefs to keep you "stuck" so that they can remain in control. Remember, the traumatic events and intense emotions you have been carrying around your whole life become beliefs, and they are real but not true *now*. The power is in the present—which is how to have FUN® and fall awake.

The following list of beliefs that are real but not true *now* can provide an even deeper look at the Committee's agenda—meaning these false beliefs may make the monkeys jump even harder. Before you look at it and find out which member of the Committee (yes, name them) makes a *special* contribution to your "being stuck," see if you can think of how these beliefs limit your life in the present.

1. I'll never be happy because I . . . .

2. I need to be perfect, and my . . . . prevents that.

3. . . . . makes me different, abnormal.

4. My . . . . limits where I can go and what I can do.

5. I'm a burden to my family and friends because of my . . . .

6. I have . . . . because my father (mother/grandparent) has it.

7. There's nothing I can do about this disease except take medication and do what the doctor says.

8. This is only going to get worse.

9. It's better not to have or enjoy sex and intimacy because . . . .

10. . . . . will shorten my life.

If you are not paying attention (*Focus*) and rewording (*Undo*) what you are saying to yourself, the story goes on and on and you will not be able to move forward (*Now what?*)—and having "fun" and living freely will not be possible in the present.

Once the client (or we) has taken an inventory of beliefs held, how do you work with them? Conventional psychotherapy tells us that "insight" will do it for us. How do we (you and your clients), you may ask, obtain this "insight?" When we (you and your clients) know and understand the "cause" of our (you and your clients') difficulty, how do we (you and your clients) "get healed," or at least feel somewhat better? Healing occurs when we become intraconnected. This, according to Siegel (2023), occurs when we fall awake. Using his Wheel of Awareness practice—being aware and open to what he refers to as "maximal uncertainty"—we can then liberate ourselves to live fully in an integrative flow of a compassionate (Monkey Mind-free) world. Knowledge is power but, in truth, it is only a brief "fix." The whole point of the brain therapies and approaches in this book is to hopefully make a mindful shift to the tools we have now to self-regulate. We can see how our beliefs can determine our responses to a situation, event, symptom, or difficulty. And when we begin to recognize and not fester in a limiting belief, we create the space necessary for contemplation about it, which, in turn, enables us to eliminate or transform it—and replace it with a new belief and a new experience.

The Space Exercise is a simple process for separating from the beliefs that create limitation. Its purpose is to detach from any chosen circumstance, item, person, belief, or event (past or present.) The only requirement for doing this exercise is that you focus (simply notice), rather than think (you can tell the neocortex-cortical "upstairs" brain that it can relax for a moment). In plain words, just be curious and give it a try, without needing an explanation, or to figure it out, or understand what this is going to do. There is no right or wrong way, no matter what the Committee members tell you (or the screaming monkeys)—it's time to go into the "downstairs" brain.

THE SPACE EXERCISE

1. Look around the room you are in right now and name or identify aloud three things/objects that you see. They could be to the left, the right, above, below, or behind you.

2. Now that you have named the three objects, look at the first one. Can you feel a *separation* between yourself and whatever it is (the computer, table, this book, a picture, the wall, ceiling, etc.)? Maybe say, "I see the picture/book/doorknob/ computer." Once you *name* or *identify* it, you differentiate from it—that is, you know you are separate from it, that it is not *you*, no matter how attached or unattached you feel to the thing.

3. Now *feel the space* between you and this object. If you stop for a moment and *focus*, or "concentrate without effort," you can definitely feel that there's space between you and the object. As you continue to focus, you may notice that you become further and further apart and that there is more room between you and the object than you first experienced.

4. Now do this again with the two remaining things that you have chosen to name. One at a time, name them, and feel the *separation* from them. Then feel the space separating you from the object by focusing or concentrating without effort.

5. Now think of a belief you hold that's negative or limiting. You can try using one of the beliefs from the belief inventory, or you may want to begin with something else, something fairly neutral. Then go through the same process again. Identify it and name it (the belief, idea, thought). Feel a separation from it. Then give yourself some space between you and it. What happens when you do this? How do you feel? What do you notice now?

Don't be discouraged if feeling a separation from an object or belief doesn't happen immediately. Detaching or separating may take practice. Using the Become an Astronaut: Put On Your Protective Space Suit or Silencing the Alarm exercises (see Chapter 8) or simple breathing exercises—such as softly inhaling the word "let" and exhaling the word "go," before you practice the Space Exercise can be helpful—try it!

Deeply held beliefs

The difficulty that can arise while doing exercises about separating or creating space from people, places, things/situations, and our beliefs is that it reveals how closely or intensely we may be attached to them. In fact, clients (or ourselves) may have certain beliefs or feel so pre-occupied by the energy of other people, places, and things that separating or creating distance from them can feel impossible. They may even report feeling tightness in various parts of the body as they try the Space Exercise on their own or during the session.

Here is where conducting, as Robin Shapiro, leading EMDR master trainer, calls it, a personectomy may work. This is where you actually "pull out" and remove the energy of the impossible person/place/thing from the client's body with your hands, very intently and fast, and then use an imaginary zipper to "zip up" the front of the client's body. Or doing an imaginary "exorcism" may also be indicated, getting out all the venom and negative energy and then filling the space cleared with an appropriate something else (blue light, warm honey, calm breeze, etc.). Then all the "refuse" that has been eliminated can be "buried" in an imaginary deep hole in the ground to the left.

As I know from experience, attachment, separation, and loss, particularly having to do with parents, are major emotional issues for people with asthma and other chronic respiratory illnesses. Many of my clients report that their initial diagnosis of asthma and other breathing difficulties appeared around the time of separation or breakups in the family: parental divorces, death of a parent, or loved ones leaving them in one way or another and being left in the care of someone else, or when they themselves were first leaving home.

> Kate had her first asthma attack at the age of three. This was shortly after her mother was diagnosed with ovarian cancer. Even though no one had discussed the possibility that her mother might die, she knew this could happen and the thought of this separation was unbearable. It was right at this time that the asthma surfaced.
>
> Another client, Carol, who is a complex trauma survivor (her father had sexually abused her for years), had trouble stabilizing her emotions and she numbed them with medication. When we did the Space Exercise, she had trouble feeling a separation from the "drama" in her head. It was as if dissociation had become her go-to way of calming herself. By depending so thoroughly on the drama, dissociation, and medication, she had no sense that there was another way to live. One of the blocking beliefs that came to light during our work was, "If I calm down and stop talking about what happened, if I enjoy my life, it means I have let him off the hook." She had held this belief for as long as she could remember. We explored her beliefs to work on possible replacements, such as: "He does not have that power over me anymore" and "He is no longer hurting me." In addition to feeling more in control and with no need for more dramatic emotions (drama no more), she told me that her family had begun remarking on how much more pleasant it was to be around her and how she seemed happier. Her story is a stunning reminder of the power of *focus*. A while later, she called to tell me her father had died and that she really was free now.

Another way to work with beliefs and help clients release the anger, rage, or troubling thoughts stored in the basement of their brain is through automatic writing. Have the client write a letter they will not send (write, not text or email). This can be a cathartic way to make what is invisible, visible. The letter can also then be brought into the therapy session to focus on using EMDR, Brainspotting, or Yoga Nidra (through sankalpa or intention setting).

When working with beliefs, the session can always end with a preferred insight that can be installed with the client doing a Butterfly Hug or a gentle tapping around the heart (whichever they prefer). I usually end these sessions with a calming exercise, such as the Container or Light Stream (see Chapter 8), so clients can leave what was worked on at my office and go out into their life less burdened (although the cortical brain will likely continue to think about what happened).

Paying attention with a nonreactive mind

My primary focus at this point on the journey in the brain forest is how to apply all the brain therapies and other methods in this book into your own life journey and/ or how to use them with your clients to know how to find and maintain a restful, nonreactive mind—no matter what is going on around us. It is challenging to stay present with what is showing up and temporarily visiting again or for the first time (anger, worry, hurt, betrayal, addiction relapse, resentment, etc.) without engaging in the reactive mind or impulsive behavior—dramatic reactions or performing is no longer needed. I refer to this as "drama no more."

A gentle warning: Even though you may find The Fun® Program (a CBT therapy), EMDR, Brainspotting, and Yoga Nidra helpful, you will be challenged on your journey and may "relapse" into old ways of thinking and "beliefing" because the Committee may think quite the contrary, telling you: "You are crazy!" or: "Therapy didn't work this other time." Or it may just say "yes" to you, and then still tell you to do it their way (all of which is okay!). Also, just because you are falling awake does not mean others will be interested in coming along to join you.

A police officer told me a story called "On Wolves, Sheep, and Sheep Dogs" (Grossman and Christensen 2004): Sheep just go with "the herd mentality" and do not make waves. Wolves are always looking for a way in to take over or attack when the sheep are not paying attention. Sheep dogs (which I am hoping you are becoming since you are reading this book), however, are both part of and outside the herd. The sheep dog is a member of this world but not of it—they participate and are staying awake and watching what is going on. When you can observe, stay awake, and be in nonreactive mode, to your family or partner you may be seen as a threat, or a "non-sheep." That is, you know how to be in the herd (it is okay to keep your head down and blend in with the sheep), but it is also important to stay awake—and know when not to be herd-like. This can happen when you go to therapy or start questioning what you thought was "normal" in your family of origin or relationship. Maybe it was normal, or a method of survival, but then it no longer "worked" or felt accurate. When you start waking up with brain therapies, you will find that waking up actually feels good!

You may think that you have abandoned the herd because you "have changed," or maybe you feel ashamed when you have joined in again. But have no fear! Trust what you are learning for yourself, and instead of asking, "What is wrong with me?" ask, "What do I want?" or, "What matters to me now?" and then, "go with that," or, "go from there," or, "be still and WAIT" (Why Am I Talking?) and see what comes. In this work, everything that occurs is welcome.

Our position from a brain therapy perspective is that "thinking" is overrated (although the neocortex can believe otherwise and try to derail the processing) and the *beliefs held* are the foundation for exploration and healing. The neocortex is like a playmate in the playground, and it is changing and demanding attention all the time. The amygdala is like an unregulated child with ADHD having a temper tantrum and the hippocampus is writing everything down in a journal—keeping a ledger—and, as we have seen, *the body is keeping the score.*

The journey of falling awake requires time to reflect, do the work of challenging beliefs held (some of them—keep the ones that work for you!), and perhaps try something different. When engaging in self-reflection, consider when, where, and with whom you seem most vulnerable or triggered, and explore these with a trained therapist, sponsor, or trusted colleague. Relapse into old ways of thinking and reacting can occur long before the unhealthy behaviors or responses to situations or people happen. It is often these habitual beliefs or engaging the Committee that led up to it. When we are not paying attention, we miss the storm warnings about a stressful situation or reaction, and before we know it, we are in the middle of a dangerous storm. Remember, *you* are not the problem—it is the story or negative beliefs you hold that are now driving the bus into that bad emotional neighborhood (stay out of the hood).

The 4 C's

In my work, I developed the "4 C's" as a reminder for staying mindfully authentic and present while on the journey of falling awake, so that we can always return to being:

- *C*onsistent: Practice daily self-care, no matter what challenges you face (you have the power over your time and focus).

- *C*urious: Be open to considering new options and possibilities.

- *C*ompassionate: Know that others may be on their own journey (don't take their responses personally), so stay true to yours.

- *C*aring: Be kind to yourself and others; we all are dealing with something.

Shifting our understanding of addiction

The 4th step of the Twelve Steps from Adult Children of Alcoholics® & Dysfunctional Families involves taking a "moral inventory." You do this by considering and writing down (getting curious about, as we learned earlier) *your* part or motive in a situation (if any)—not to create blame, just to be awake to and look squarely at the unhappiness you may have created for yourself and others. This can often be linked back to the "normal" you grew up in or that was caused by something that occurred in the past. According to Leela (2022) and Marich and Dansinger (2022), the Twelve

Steps program proposes that by uncovering your emotional attachments and your drama belief network, you can move toward correcting them; without doing this, you can't experience genuine sobriety (emotional or abstinence), contentment, and peace of mind. Adult Children of Alcoholics® & Dysfunctional Families refer to it as "becoming your own loving parent." Expectations, resentments, and bitter feelings can create the perfect circumstances for us to become victims again in that we no longer feel obliged or able to work toward healing, choosing instead to identify with our pain ("Poor me" or "Pour me a drink" or "I'm going to eat some cake"). Yet, as unwholesome as this can be, this state of feeling helpless is also a *natural visitor* of our emotional palette. When we acknowledge that it is okay to be upset as a natural response to what is going on right now, we reconnect with our hurt in a constructive way and can begin again the process of falling and remaining awake. We now have some tools to work through it and we use them!

Alcoholism, addiction, and family dysfunction, as opposed to the medical disease model, are now considered by many to be ways of coping as a result of a combination of very complex circumstances that can include culture, politics, religion, domestic violence, death, divorce, sexual trauma, bullying, caregiver neglect, generational trauma, and/or plain old family "rules," rather than that we are engaged in bad habits or are defective in some way. You can use the Impact of Events Scale or the ACE Questionnaire to assess the possible origins of your or your client's current addictions and dysfunctions. More importantly, we look at these behaviors to understand the ways in which we experience suffering: It's not how much you use alcohol, drugs, or smoke weed; it's what happens when you do. What does the using offer? How did it become "normal" to establish ourselves in this behavior/dysfunction?

In addition to exploring our addiction(s) with brain therapies, we, or our clients, may benefit from the support of Adult Children of Alcoholics® & Dysfunctional Families, Alcoholics Anonymous (AA), Al-Anon, or other 12-step programs, as these self-help organizations, freely available world-wide, offer health and hope to millions of recovering alcoholics and people impacted by dysfunctional family patterns. These programs support the ongoing awareness that your sobriety, recovery, and peace of mind require *taking responsibility for the consequences of your actions/behavior*—and that you can do this only by first looking inward at the beliefs, desires, and thoughts that govern your actions. This is in no way blaming you for your actions, beliefs, or behavior. However, it is important to be curious about how all these ways of coping developed in order to become your own authority, unattached to old, unhealthy beliefs and stories and eventually, free from the damaging impact of the past.

Our minds have a tendency to convince us that certain thoughts are of the utmost importance and that we need to act immediately because of them. Once we are aware that our thinking is not always helpful or useful, we can more easily calm the impending feeling storm that may be forming in our brain forest. When we notice what we are "thinking," thoughts have less power over us. As a result, we can make decisions that are based on our true intention and motives. Remembering that nothing is as critical as we are beliefing it to be (unless there is actual danger) calms the brainbody, and life begins to seem lighter as we drop our baggage (try relaxing your shoulders as you read this—that's the feeling!).

I hope by now you are learning how important it is to work with your beliefs, and that when the storms of life temporarily put you to the test (emotionally, psychologically, physically, and/or spiritually), brain therapies can help you to stay present, quiet the mind, and relax the body. It is our responsibility to choose how we ride out the storm.

CHAPTER 7

What It Takes to Fall and Remain Awake

When I began my personal work with Dr. Gerald Epstein (see Chapter 1), both the imagery and his frank questioning shocked me into my first coherent experiences of the "purpose" of my symptoms and diagnosis. I discovered that my physical feeling of suffocation (asthma) mirrored the emotional suffocation I felt in the relationship I was in at that time and the circumstances in my infancy when I was diagnosed at the age of 15 months. I became aware that my constricted breathing reflected the constricting circumstances at the various stages of my life. Most importantly, the symptoms revealed that I needed to make a change in my thinking and behaviors—I needed to fall awake.

When I searched my heart for the core belief that prevented me from breaking free from the constriction and suffocation, I was dismayed to find that I believed I was unlovable. Since it's love that "makes the world go round," believing I was unlovable was literally making my entire life "unlivable." Thus, my confession to Dr. Epstein that I secretly wanted to die made a lot of sense, since "breath is life" and being asthmatic was the perfect physical mirror of my emotional and mental malaise. Dr. Epstein told me that if I wanted to heal from asthma, I had to choose to live.

What do you want to do with the brain therapies? How will using them help (have an intention or focus)?

Whether you are a therapist working on yourself or with a client or an individual beginning to explore these brain therapies, all the practices presented in this book and reviewed in this chapter can help you to stay anchored in the present. Remember the question to keep in mind always: What do you want?

Here is what you can do to *make shift happen*:

- Calm the anxious busy mind to land in the present moment and notice sensations in the body.

- Discover with curiosity and openness new options for ways of thinking and behaving, as trauma and stressful events often make people feel trapped (attached to their story).

- Create a caring, compassionate understanding and friendship with the body, mind, intense emotions, and the Committee (what is the message they are telling you?).

- Discover how beliefs become stories and how to use intention as a powerful tool for focus to stay anchored in the present.

- Understand how to activate the neural network to release stored trauma memories and process sensations and emotions energetically so the brain and nervous system can reset.

- Occupy and live safely in the brainbody right now.

How to decide which therapy to use

First, remember to always trust your clinical judgment as your clients were coming and keep coming to therapy to work with you long before you learned about the methods described in this book. Next, always obtain informed consent for the intervention you want to use, and always start with where the client is. If you have been primarily a talk therapist or have "done a lot of work" on yourself in therapy, experiencing the brainbody therapies for the first time can feel like never having been in a swimming pool before, and now you are going to jump off the diving board into the water, taking the plunge. Know that taking baby steps or starting with dipping your big toe in the water is always "okay." Falling and staying awake takes time. Honor the journey, adjust the speed, and stop to rest and reflect when you need.

However you and/or your clients decide how to begin the healing journey is absolutely correct. There is no right or wrong to do or experience what happens in any therapy or healing practice, only your way—as long as you know why you are doing what you are doing with them and what the intention is. What do you/they want?

As we have seen, with each of the brain therapies (The FUN® Program, EMDR, Brainspotting, and Yoga Nidra), we don't need to or know what's going to be released or when; we just stay curious the whole time. Remember, the most important question to ask yourself and answer is: "Why am I choosing the therapy/technique/intervention I am using for myself/with this client?" That is the question you need to be able to answer (otherwise arrange for a consultation or obtain further training).

Once you have that clarity, here is a guide for the treatment planning process with a client, no matter which of the therapies you want to use.

1. Always obtain signed or verbal informed consent.

2. All the therapies start with the setup or focus for the session: What brought the client to you? What do they want?

3. What is most important for today? Or, if the client arrives to the session activated, triggered, or very upset, ask if they would like to open this up—what is it that they would like to feel relief from or gain insight about?

4. What emotions do they feel? What is the worst belief they have about themselves as they think about this now? And what emotions are connected to this?

5. Ask the client: "How intense or activated do you feel about this *now*, on a scale of 0–10?" (0 = not at all to 10 = a lot) (Optional; this is called taking a Subjective Units of Distress Scale (SUDS) rating; see Chapter 3 and 4.)

6. What would they prefer to believe about themselves as they think about this, and how true does this feel right now? Rate the Validity of Cognition (VoC) on a scale of 1–7, one being not believable at all to seven being absolutely true (optional) (see Chapter 3).

7. Location/cue to physical sensations: As they think about this, where do they feel it in their body?

8. Allow what is coming to come, what is going to go...all is welcome here.

9. Trust what comes up or does not (there is no right or wrong, they are not here to please the therapist).

10. Bring the session to a close: Be sure to allow time for closure.

11. Install what was helpful, or calm place, perhaps by using the Container or Light Stream exercises (see Chapter 8).

When considering which therapy to use

As you think about using The FUN® Program, EMDR, Brainspotting, and/or Yoga Nidra for your clients, here are a few things to help guide you in which is best for what:

- Each of the therapies utilizes both the top-down and bottom-up approach to accessing memories and trapped emotions in the brain. And all of them energetically calm the alarm center—the amygdala and sympathetic nervous system—simultaneously.

- All the therapies encourage both top-down and bottom-up regulation—from the neck up and down. The whole body is involved by doing a body scan and noticing sensations (tightness, stiffness, butterflies/anxiety, feeling hot or cold) in that part of the body (Lusk 2021; Lutz 2021; Pyles *et al.* 2021).

- The FUN® Program, EMDR, Brainspotting, and Yoga Nidra exercises can be applied both for daily self-regulation and when triggered.

- Everybody can benefit from these techniques—unless they are under the influence of drugs or alcohol or have a psychotic mood disorder (self-reflection and insight that are not regulated). Always trust your clinical judgment and be clear about why you are doing what you are doing with a client.

- Take advanced trainings and attend workshops and conferences to be up-to-date on the latest research for treating trauma and stress-related disorders.

- Use these practices to keep yourself, and your clients, in the present moment—the past is not as important as we *believe* it to be. Remember, when you use resourcing exercises with your clients, you are also resourcing yourself.

- All brainbody skills are like a tuning fork. They polish vagal nerve tone to improve resiliency—calming the alarm center of the amygdala, relaxing muscles, quieting the mind, calming the heart, slowing the breath, improving sleep, increasing confidence.

- All these somatic therapies can stabilize the autonomic nervous system to reduce anxiety and depression and teach clients (and us) how to be in control when chronic stress reactions occur.

- All can increase positive experiences in trauma survivors by gaining new awareness, insight, and shifts in beliefs (stories), and as they learn that they probably did the best they could, given the circumstances.

- The strategies and self-soothing skills involved in brain therapies (the mind maintains a ledger) and increased knowledge of how the body keeps the score (explaining body mechanics that may go beyond the scope of this book) helps to discharge pent-up energy in the nervous system and restore a resting baseline. The mind and the body get a mental "unplug" and "reset."

- Encourage your clients to consider whether they feel this type of treatment is appropriate for them. Let the client know how to "stop" the process when they want to or if other issues come up—they are always in charge.

- How a session is opened and closed is very important. We always want the client (and ourselves) to feel at a good place to stop for the moment when the session is over.

Distinctions to consider when using The FUN® Program, EMDR, Brainspotting, and Yoga Nidra

All these brain therapies have applications that are therapeutic, and the reasons why people seek out a specific practice are similar. But there are some distinct differences.

Physical position

- The FUN® Program, EMDR, and Brainspotting are typically done in a seated position, such as on a chair, where the body is comfortable, yet upright and alert. EMDR is conducted by a licensed mental health professional. Brainspotting does not require licensure by a mental health professional, but formal training by Brainspotting International is required. Yoga Nidra is usually done lying on the ground, preferably on a yoga mat, but can also be done seated in a chair. Yoga teacher training (YTT), and training specifically in Yoga Nidra, is highly recommended. Yoga Nidra training is best when done by a certified yoga instructor who has trauma-informed training. You do not need to be a mental health professional to learn and offer Yoga Nidra sessions.

- During the FUN® therapy session and other talk therapies, what may be chosen by the client to be "processed" is a current stressor or critical incident in the present or a past trauma that is being reexperienced due to recent stressors that are engaging the fight, flight, freeze, or faint response. Psychoeducation is offered and The FUN® Program is provided to learn how beliefs and ways of thinking are accelerating the stress response.

- To prepare for, and during, the EMDR session, the client consciously places their attention on the bilateral stimulation (BLS) chosen (eye movements, tapping, tappers, headphones, etc.). Once the issue that brought them to the session has been determined, or something else has been chosen as the focus to work on, it is then determined how intense or activated they feel about it right now (Bae and Kim 2012). As you think about this incident/problem/issue on a scale from 0–10, where 0 is no activation, disturbance, or neutral, to 10 being the highest disturbance you can imagine, how activated or upset does this feel to you right now? Negative and preferred cognitions associated with the target as well as body sensations may be explored. Then, whatever comes up during EMDR processing, the therapist instructs the client to "go with that."

- A similar process occurs with Brainspotting, except once the issue to work on has been determined and how intense or activated they are about it now (on a scale from 0–10), and where they feel this in their body, the "brainspot" (where the intense memories may be stored) is discovered by using a pointer or watching where the eyes go and get activated (blinking, facial expressions, body movements, etc.). Once the activation or brainspot is determined, the practitioner "holds the spot" (with the pointer, or gazespot, and optional bilateral music on headphones). Then the practitioner applies the acronym WAIT (Why Am I Talking?), to "see" what comes to conscious awareness. Different responses may be used when the client shares what is happening, such as "There is information there, just go from there" or "Be curious about that and see what comes up." Neither EMDR nor Brainspotting engages in questions or providing feedback during processing. We want to stay in the subcortical brain.

- During Yoga Nidra, the client gets into a relaxed, usually reclining position (on their back, side or stomach—whatever is most comfortable) on the floor on a yoga mat/towel/blanket (seated in a chair is also okay, with the back resting against a wall so they can rest the head if they want) with the eyes closed, and is taken on a guided imaginary journey around the body into deeper states of consciousness (beta, gamma, alpha, theta, delta; see Desai 2017, p.36). No talking or movement is required or necessary. Emotions, thoughts, and memories may come to consciousness (real or imagined, like a dream state), and then be released.

- During processing in all these methods, questions and discussion can cautiously be addressed just before the session and are gently shut down as we do not want the cortical analytical brain to get involved (engage the Committee, etc.). Debriefing can occur after all these sessions; however, the client is encouraged to let the brain continue processing what happened and bring back what they notice (dreams, memories, revelations, etc.) to the next session to continue the work. Any of the resourcing discussed in this and subsequent chapters can be encouraged for the client to use after or between sessions if there is activation or triggers. (Dr. Francine Shapiro's TICES (Trigger, Image, Cognition, Emotions, Sensation) can be helpful here; Shapiro 2007; see also Appendix E.)

State of consciousness

- In EMDR, Brainspotting, and Yoga Nidra, people can experience multiple states of consciousness within a single session. Many will remain in what is known as the waking state of consciousness (beta, the active and alert mind experience that occurs in talk therapy), which is the frame of mind most of us spend our waking hours in. The mindfulness that can occur during brain therapies are the techniques that take you and your clients into different levels of consciousness (alpha, theta, etc.) and even beyond—into the deepest levels of relaxation when the mind may go offline (delta), and experience deep healing and restorative sleep—such as the state of falling awake.

What can occur in an EMDR, Brainspotting, and Yoga Nidra session

What happens when using the FUN® Program, EMDR, Brainspotting, or during a Yoga Nidra session depends on the client (age, stage of recovery in addiction, supports in place, motivation, informed consent, etc.) and level/location of care (residential, outpatient clinic, private practice other clinical setting) or a yoga studio. All these practices take place in diverse settings and have a different "culture" which may impact the choice to participate. The following are basic guidelines for you to consider to make your setting inclusive, integrative, and trauma-informed:

- Psychoeducation: Going back to the first session exercise: What do they want today? And which practice would they like to use to open this up (obtaining informed consent).

- Creating and securing the space for healing: Connecting with the person while obtaining client history and treatment planning (new to these practices, presenting problem, determining their window of tolerance, etc.).

- Preparation: Issue to work on today (setting an intention).

- Assessment: Clinical judgment if/what may be appropriate to use (including just talk therapy, The FUN® Program, etc.), notice their breathing, body posture, eye gazing, facial expression, nervous system activation (a SUDS may be taken here).

- Desensitization: Holding the secure, confidential space to release intense feelings, memories, emotions.

- Installation/resourcing: What do they want to remember that was helpful about the session (new insights, cognitions, ways of thinking, etc.).

- Body scan: What are they sensing in the body now?

- Closure: Encourage the use of resources learned (calming exercises).

- Debriefing/reevaluation: Ask about insights, new thoughts, a reminder that the brain will keep processing. Keep notes/a journal to discuss at the next session.

Benefits of The FUN® Program, EMDR, Brainspotting, and Yoga Nidra

All the brain therapies as well as talk therapy can be about accessing, dismantling, and properly processing highly charged emotions, negative beliefs, and stories from clients' lives that may be keeping them stuck. It is the present focus (making use of the neurophysiology discussed in this book) that unlocks stored information that may not be accessible in the traditional talk therapies—when words cannot express or describe the activation they feel.

Please remember, the rapid bilateral eye movements of EMDR, the eye gaze/brainspot in Brainspotting, and the relaxing introspection of Yoga Nidra can put a spotlight on the intense emotions, beliefs, and memories related to a trauma or incident that occurred and reveal life situations to reflect on from a detached perspective—like watching a movie on a blank screen. They all can be helpful to relieve charged emotional states: anxiety, anger, panic, sleep disturbance, guilt, resentment, and shame—which all may be linked to disturbing memories or negative beliefs created from the past or in anticipation of the future—and it may happen more than once...hence single session therapy is rare.

Clients diagnosed with chronic health issues, PTSD, trauma, addiction, eating disorders, and other mood disturbances have reported the following benefits from EMDR, Brainspotting, and Yoga Nidra:

- Calming the central nervous system

- Increasing the knowledge and ability to self-soothe

- Improving sleep

- Regaining a sense of control during and between sessions

- Decreasing anxiety

- Alleviating stress

- Finding peace with changes in appearance (aging), and body image (eating disorders, cancer surgery, etc.)

- More control over PTSD reactions and symptoms

- Reducing addictive cravings

- Addressing fears and beliefs about life and death

- Transforming beliefs, behaviors, and ways of thinking

- Fostering feelings of peace, calm, and clarity.

How to get started...

Here are some examples of techniques or strategies you may already know or can try (and make them your own). You create the secure space, provide the energy, and that felt sense of belonging and being welcome in the confidential session. The is done with attunement to your attentive, regulated, and alert presence in your office (live or virtual):

- Transformational, attentive, inclusive language is always key, whether you are working with trauma, attachment, neglect, betrayal, anxiety, or depression, along with kind, considerate communication (tone of voice can make a huge impact). For example (in live sessions at the office), in FUN®, EMDR, and Brainspotting sessions, distance from the client, and where you are sitting during the session, placement of hands in front of the face for EMDR or the pointer during Brainspotting is important to establish up front (for virtual sessions too). During Yoga Nidra, you might say, "Please place the legs about shoulder width apart (or as wide as your yoga mat)." Or, "Relax" instead of, "Hang the head." Have clients "expand the chest" (instead of "open the chest and heart") "and notice the breath in front of and at the back of or behind the heart...notice your heart beat." You can also say, "Inhale, 'I am,' exhale 'here,'" or, "Breathe in health, exhale what no longer serves you," or, "Inhale sober calm, exhale and release all the restrictions, obstacles, inner weapons of mass destruction," or, "Inhale 'let,' exhale, 'go,'" or simply, "See and inhale the word 'peace,' and exhale 'peace.'"

- When treating a trauma, and in all clinical settings, we are always sensitive and attentive to language, culture, religion, race, and gender. We are inclusive, not exclusive. What we say and how we say it *always* matters. We integrate trauma-sensitive practices in all clinical behavioral healthcare—everyone is coming to you because *something happened or is happening to them.*

- During Brainspotting watch where the eyes go, where they find "the spot." This is the location of the brainspot where the client feels or seems most activated. There is no "right spot." There may be several where they can keep their gaze while information from the brain is activated and accessed for processing in the session. You may say, "We trust your brainbody and eyes know, as 'where you look affects how you feel.'"

- During an EMDR session, clients often ask: "Which works the best: the tappers, the horizontal eye movements, bilateral sound, or tapping for processing?" We might say, "What would you like to try first? Let's try that and go from there." Also, when using your hand for BLS, be attuned to where you sit (it is suggested to sit on a client's left so you have the heart-to-heart connection), and establish how close you sit.

- Remember to have fun with FUN®...here shift happens...and stop taking everything so seriously! Unless you are in danger, you may need to lighten the load! Remember, drama no more... We want your ventral vagal system to be able to make decisions (Chapter 1). Try befriending the Committee and the brainbody—The Shamer, The Inner Critic, The Protector, The Perfectionist—as they are your defense mechanisms and have been created by you for a reason—at the time you needed them. We honor, love, respect, and care for all these "parts" of you, including all "parts" of the body: front/back, upper/lower, right/left, feet, face, etc. They have all made their presence known to you at that time in your life; they just may need to back off and go on vacation. These parts may show up and visit from time to time to "see" if they are needed. Remember, you are in charge *now.* This is the essence of The FUN® Program. Are you sick and tired of being sick and tired? If not now, when? You can't do it alone, but you alone must do it (don't let the Committee run your life!).

- Tools for self-soothing are portable and always available. Using the brainbody therapies and yoga therapeutically is about being at home, being present in your mind and body—the lights are on when you are falling awake and paying attention.

- Trauma/crisis/pain/overwhelm/flashback/dissociation is about not being in the present or in the brainbody. It's like driving home and not remembering what route you took or missing the turn. You just somehow "got there," driving at 85 mph on automatic pilot. Or walking into the kitchen and not remembering why you went in there. Usually, we keep acting like this until the shit hits the fan. Yoga is about being in the body and noticing all sensations, feelings, wrinkles, flab, etc. Addiction is about being in the body artificially. Yoga is being in the present in the brainbody.

- Brainbody practices equal attention. Focus, intention, obsessive thinking, and beliefs put pressure on the neural pathways of the brain and nervous system. The brainbody therapies are breaking the habit of distraction and numbing out. We have the DNA to move away from the past. We are always thinking about something. When we are falling awake, we are paying attention and can decide if this way of thinking is helping, or if we need to intervene using the practices in the book and/or with a therapist.

Remember, in addition to the inner work…you've got to move. To heal from illness and dis-ease (stress/tension) there must be movement, otherwise falling awake has stopped and we become stuck. Here are some suggestions that can easily be done by you and your clients (together) in and during sessions (and as homework between sessions):

- An easy overhead stretch (like picking apples), arm swings, and shoulder rolls: This opens the chest, back, and heart to increase energy, balance moods, and change posture—even just relaxing the shoulders away from the ears can create a shift.

- Breath of joy/conduct the orchestra: This boosts mood, reduces fatigue and depression, and distracts looping in the busy mind. Here's how to do it (for more details and other similar exercises, see Weintraub 2012, pp.80–83). Stand with feet shoulder width apart and parallel, knees slightly bent, as though you are about to sit in a chair. Inhale one-third of your lung capacity through the nostrils as you swing the arms up in front of the body until they are parallel to each other at shoulder level. Continue inhaling to two-thirds capacity and stretch the arms out to the side like wings at shoulder level. Inhale to full capacity and swing the arms parallel and over the head, palms facing each other. Open the mouth and exhale completely with an audible "ha," bending the knees more deeply as you sink into a standing squat, and swing the arms down and back behind you like a diver, palms facing in. Repeat several times (5–9) at a moderate pace without forcing or straining the body or breath. Simply pay attention and be absorbed by the peaceful, relaxing rhythm. Then return to standing, close the eyes, and notice the efforts of breath of joy. Feel the sensations in the face and arms and the tingling in the hands and fingers.

- Moving marching stomps in place: This helps to build and increase a sense of control in the body and can release tension. It can be done live or virtually.

- Elbow to knee, leg swings, shake it out, bounce, hula hip circles: This encourages balance in the body, which can be difficult for trauma survivors because of changes in their nervous system.

- Shake it off: Like the song American singer-songwriter Taylor Swift (1989) recorded, make a noise, then be still and just notice.

Clients may think this is silly or that they are "paying you so they can talk," but just encourage them to try (informed consent) just one of these with you, and see how they feel in your office now!

Tools for crisis situations—no certification required!

How do we respond to crisis or extreme overwhelm? What are the protocols for immediate relief in a traumatic, highly stressful, or dangerous situation? One approach is called critical incident debriefing (CID), developed by Roy Kiessling. Here is how he explained it to me (direct communication, May 1, 2023):

> As an EMDR clinician, I have always admired the ability of eye movements and other distracting activities (DAS, dual attention stimulation) in rapidly reducing levels of disturbance and emotional activation. However, sometimes during an EMDR session, pre-existing issues unrelated to the presenting crisis can become activated. For processing recent events, this has become a real concern.
>
> Within the EMDR community, revisions of EMDR have been developed to use in diverse settings. However, these interventions are restricted to only those trained in EMDR. Only Master's level or above licensed clinicians are eligible to be trained in EMDR; thus, only they are eligible to use EMDR-related recent event protocols.
>
> My first exposure to the need to provide a crisis intervention that was not considered EMDR was in 1998 when I traveled to Bangladesh. Only psychiatrists and psychologists were eligible to be trained in EMDR; however, many well-educated individuals were running non-governmental organizations (NGOs) dealing with severely traumatized clients who could have benefited from some type of crisis intervention.
>
> From that experience, it became one of my missions to develop a brief, safe, and effective crisis intervention that could address clients in crisis while not being considered EMDR. CID is the final product. We wanted to create something like the Heimlich maneuver, which is not a medical procedure, for a person who is choking, something that can be used to save their life. In many respects, CID is the Heimlich Maneuver for someone "psychologically" choking on an emotionally "choking" experience.

Distracting activities, whether it be eye movements, physical tapping, progress counting, or an iPhone app, cause emotions to become less intense, independent of any relationship or preexisting psychological history. In other words, it does not require taking a history or establishing a diagnosis. As such, CID is positioned as a crisis intervention independent of EMDR or traditional talk therapy.

Since 2013, CID has gone through various modifications, mainly to refine the procedures so they can be used by anyone (much like the Heimlich maneuver for someone choking). CID has been taught to police and law enforcement professionals, emergency medical technicians, firefighters, lay professionals, volunteers, as well as the general public.

Most recently, Kiessling and his team have expanded CID into the virtual environment. He has collaborated with a group in the Netherlands (Moovd) to develop a self-contained iPhone/Android app that creates the CID protocols without any additional training while also providing the stimulation in a managed way, that is, stimulating without over-accessing. The virtual app can be accessed through Moovd, known as Moovment—a 24/7 emergency tool when the amygdala's smoke detector goes off (see Chapter 1).

The CID protocol

Here is the simple procedure to be followed, once connection/attunement and rapport has been established:

1. What is the problem? What happened? (If the client is too dysregulated, this step may be skipped.)

2. How disturbing is it on a scale of 0–10? (SUDS)

3. Distracting stimulation, that is, eye movements, rapid tapping (arms crossed butterfly tapping, tapping on the biceps), counting (backwards, subtracting by 7 from 100), etc. for roughly 5–10 seconds.

4. How disturbing is it now, using the same 0–10 scale? (SUDS)

5. Repeat steps 3 and 4 until the disturbance is decreasing.

It is important to stop the stimulation if the disturbance begins to increase, which may indicate a more deeply seated traumatic experience is being activated. Should that occur, we recommend seeking a licensed mental health professional (or EMDR/Brainspotting therapist) to explore and treat these connections. That's the protocol.

CID is more focused on the immediate trauma—for example, to use on the scene as a first responder or when you see clients soon after an incident. When used after the impact of a trauma, it is less likely that pre-existing issues (that feel or seem similar to the storage in the brainstem) will become activated. CID can be used initially in a clinical session when clients arrive activated or on the scene of a trauma. CID can also be used to provide immediate relief from the overwhelm of the trauma. This relief can lay the groundwork to shift to other interventions for processing—later, or after the nervous system has calmed down.

Here is an EMDR-"related intervention" (CID) that anyone can use—no EMDR certification required.

Nancy (a complex trauma client I have been seeing for several years) arrived late to my office for her appointment, yelling at her husband on her cell phone and very activated. She was furious with him, as he had stained the bathtub in her home, and was crying hysterically and showing me pictures of the tub on her cell phone.

> He doesn't understand how much I do around the house trying to fix it up! [They had recently moved into a rental.] I am trying to decorate, we have shit in boxes everywhere, what does he expect of me? I can't help it if I have thick hair that backs up the drain.

Having learned CID, I used CID. Nancy said her SUDS was a 7 and that she felt hot and sweaty all over her body. We were tapping on our forearms together while she provided the details of her aggravation. Just using CID for the entire session to calm her down, by the end she said she felt a lot calmer and light (SUDS between a 2 and a 3). We shut the session down by her sensing the lightness she felt in her chest now, and she shared that she associated the calmness with the color blue. She called me later to let me know she was much better and was heading to a yoga class at the beach. She also shared that she had downloaded the Moovment app on her phone, which mimics the CID we used together in the session. This "on-demand" EMDR tool she can use if she gets upset and aggravated again.

This is also an example which illustrates that we don't need to get all the details up front—our task is to help our clients self-regulate while they tell their story. Between the sets of BLS, she shared other things that she was upset about, like she was changing the TV channels with the remote, moving between the "History" channel and the "Discovery" channel. Here the alarm center (amygdala) was starting to shift from chaos to calm. During this, she made the connection (in the "History" channel) that the current stressor, and her intense responses and reactions to her husband, lit up memories about "no one paying attention" to her needs and not feeling cared about in her childhood.

"Stopped at the red light, I wish I had kept going"[1]

I work part time in a hospital setting and recently have had many opportunities to utilize BLS as a calming tool. One recent incident involved an elderly couple who were getting ready for church on a Sunday morning. The husband began experiencing chest pains and they got in the car and headed for the ER. He had been in the ER the week before and was told he was having a panic attack and was sent home. But this time, he told his wife, felt different. They were stopped at a red light directly in front of the hospital within sight of the ER when the husband began gurgling and slumped over in his seat. The wife could not make herself run the red light and so sat for a few minutes with her husband making these sounds.

Upon arrival at the ER, her husband was swept into the treatment room (he had died in the car), and she was left in the hallway alone with the intent of calling her children. I was called to come be with her, as she was too upset to make calls

---

1 This case was shared by Angela Gingerich, LCSW, EMDR practitioner.

or even to speak. When I arrived at the ER, she was tearful, rocking and mumbling incoherently. I was able to establish eye contact and ask her permission to "try something." She said "sure," and I led her through Silencing the Alarm and several rounds of CID. These two tools enabled her to stop shaking, use her phone to call her children and speak coherently. In CID, her SUDS was reduced from a 10 to a 4. When her family arrived, her daughter-in-law began experiencing a panic attack. The wife asked if I could "do that thing" with her daughter-in-law and we engaged in CID related to flashbacks the daughter-in-law was experiencing in relation to her own heart attack two years earlier. Several of the family members had questions about "what did you do?" and asked many questions about EMDR, CID, and BLS in general, and expressed gratitude for the availability of these tools.

Combining CID and EMDR, talk therapy, or another trauma intervention

After the shooting at the 4th of July parade in Highland Park, Illinois, in 2022, the use of CID was integrated with other trauma methods by EMDR clinicians who came to the scene as part of the trauma response team. The following is an example of how CID was integrated, along with challenges experienced, to process the critical incident (as reported to Roy Kiessling, direct communication, edited and told with permission by Corrie Goldberg 2022):

> The EMDR clinicians were sent to a high school cafeteria to provide crisis coun-selling for people who had been at the parade and for those not at the parade but impacted by the incident. The trauma therapists were volunteers from the community with diverse specializations. The EMDR clinicians who volunteered to help shared that they had reviewed the CID video prior to going and brought the pocket "cheat sheets" with them to stay focused and refrain from getting triggered by the stories they would hear.
>
> The therapists were at the school Friday evening and all day Saturday, as it took time to really "grasp" the full scope of what was going on. The cafeteria was crowded, with lots of noise and distractions around them, including therapy dogs, children, FBI agents in black vests, volunteer "ambassadors" in yellow vests, translators (for those who spoke only Spanish) in green vests, Red Cross volunteers in white vests, and a squeaky door that made a sound like a dog (or a child) whimpering every time it was opened or closed.
>
> The people they worked with were masked [it was during the Covid-19 pan-demic], red-eyed, and teary. Those who spoke Spanish were provided with a volun-teer translator. Since the therapist had no information prior to working with them (Were they at the parade or not? Had they spoken to other volunteers already?), they just launched into the CID protocol and asked the person to tell them what had happened (again, the details are not that important at this moment—this was just to facilitate self-regulation). One individual started to share their story through the translator, but became visibly more activated.
>
> When they seemed to struggle, getting more activated and upset, the EMDR

therapists stopped at this point and transitioned to a series of resourcing (calming) exercises to help them get grounded and stabilize, etc.

After they reported feeling calmer and could talk about what happened, the therapists continued CID, using the tapping of hands on their thighs for the BLS (they modeled the pace by watching the therapist tapping on themselves on the thighs gently while they tapped on theirs). Sometimes the therapist will ask the client who is very activated to walk around or move their feet in place while describing the event being worked on (Berceli 2005). This method of BLS was chosen because each person appeared uncomfortable with the closeness required for eye movements (sitting side by side). Although they kept reporting that they felt increasingly better with each round of BLS, they also kept stating that their SUDS remained at a 7 throughout all the processing, which may have been a function of the language barrier.

Once they said that they were feeling "much better," the therapist moved on to closure by asking how else they could help right now, and provided some of the available handouts (in Spanish) for additional counseling resources in the community. The volunteers were not sure where they went after this initial crisis stabilization session.

If the history of the people they were working with revealed past traumas that had been reactivated by this event, they did not do any EMDR active processing of any kind. If it seemed appropriate, they provided psychoeducation about EMDR as one of many trauma treatments that might be helpful to them as they worked to process this event and discussed the apparent interconnectedness of their trauma history. It was then suggested that they seek out longer-term care to do that work. At this point the EMDR therapists worked with them more on resourcing (stabilization) and psychoeducation about trauma, as well as addressed any concerns that they had about others (e.g., parents often had questions about how to support their children through this).

This is what a client at the parade reported about how EMDR had helped her:

As a result of that one-hour session, I went from feeling on high alert, unable to focus, unable to sleep, having strange dreams, startling easily, etc., etc., to suddenly being able to sense myself calming down...at least sometimes. Since then, I've had two more sessions with her, and we have slowly done desensitization (BLS) on the worst parts of that day.

What my therapist said would happen is starting to happen—I'm able to be calmer and not have my mental state taken over by the fear [what she called "being hijacked by the amygdala," where the part of the brain that controls emotions goes into overdrive when thinking about the traumatic incident, even if no actual danger is present anymore]. EMDR has by no means taken away the horror and the fear and the awfulness of the shooting. It has by no means made it "okay," whatever that would mean, and my heart is still broken and breaking for the people in this town and what they are going through. And although I'm still having strange dreams—some of them more explicitly related to the actual events now that we're a week or two out—still, sometimes I start to feel my heart race when I think about what I went through. I can also simply think about what happened and process it without being totally taken over by it, and that's good and necessary progress.

Other factors learned while helping at this tragedy

From a demographic diversity perspective, the therapists on site reported that a significant percentage of those affected were Latinos (from many Hispanic origins), Orthodox Jewish individuals, Native Americans, LBGTQIA+ people, or from other ethnic, racial, religious, tribal neighborhoods. Many of these community members had lived in the area or town for years or decades, having multigenerational ties to the area where the shooting occurred. Prior traumas that seemed to be activated by this event included direct experiences with other mass shootings or acts of terrorism (in their community, university, at an event, etc.) or being a member of minority group targeted in other mass shootings, acts of terrorism, or hate crimes.

Other considerations

- One individual found tapping hands on the thighs, a form of BLS, activating, as the sound of tapping the legs reminded them of the sound of the gunshots, so they switched to Butterfly Hug.

- The sounds, activity, etc. in the environment were activating to many of the people present because the events at the parade involved a lot of startling noise, sounds of people, and a flurry of activity. This was a challenging factor, given the setting.

- Many who were impacted were immigrants, and these individuals were encouraged to access services regardless of immigration status. Walking into the building with federal agents everywhere could activate other trauma or stress.

- Although not technically "at the parade," several park district employees/camp counselors, who were mostly teenagers, were assigned to work at the festival at the park that marked the end of the parade route. These individuals were under lockdown in a small building at the park and were then reportedly released to walk back to their cars or walk home shortly after the shooting occurred. They may have had a more heightened trauma response than the average individual labeled as "not at the parade," so therapists working with individuals in the "not at the parade" area may want to listen for this in responding to a crisis—as this is when location does not matter—they were still impacted.

What we wear matters too

EMDR therapists were initially asked to dress in "soft colors." It appears that the colors red, royal blue, as well as white, in combination with either red or blue, had reportedly been activating to some of those affected by the shooting at the parade. In awareness of attunement, our office, showing up on site, wherever the intervention takes place, what we say, how we look, and how we respond does matter!

Trauma self-care interventions for you and/or your clients

Now let's pause and reflect for a moment here. Take some long, slow exhalations and notice what thoughts, sensations, reactions, or triggers you may have experienced just reading about this tragic incident and the interventions that were applied. During case consultation, some consultees reported being anxious about trying these techniques for fear of doing it wrong, getting distracted and thinking about other things (incidents it reminded them of, recalling hearing about it on the news), or they noticed feeling irritated, angry, or felt a strong sensation in their body (knots in the stomach, tight shoulders, etc.). These reactions that can occur for therapists are *normal* and are often referred to as vicarious traumatization or limbic countertransference.

GROUNDING PRACTICE TO RELAX AND FOCUS

How do your clients experience being in their body? Can they identify, notice, and describe sensations (not feelings) present in their bodies? Some complex trauma survivors can only describe what they "feel" from the neck up (emotions). Our job as brainbody therapists is to provide education and engage the whole body in the healing experience. (I have a client constantly tell me he does not know what that means—he can't feel anything except "right here" [points to his heart]. We start from there.) We are helping clients put into language the emotions and memories that have been activated.

This is a resourcing exercise to assess the client's window of tolerance. The interpersonal elegance of this practice can be easily applied to your way of doing therapy by just cueing sensation (and demonstrating by doing it with your client):

Notice the breath (place hands on the stomach and chest as you breathe and expand the belly and the rib cage); sense the left hand, the right hand; place both feet on the floor; notice where you are looking, close the eyes, soften the gaze, relax the shoulders.

All of these can work (with adjustments or modifications) with trauma survivors, stabilizing those in recovery from addiction, for impulse control, stabilizing moods, calming hyperarousal, or just taking a moment to "land" in the session in your office—arriving and staying in present-focused awareness.

DRAWING THE SYMPTOM/ISSUE/TRIGGER—AND SCRIBBLE IT OUT

This is a simple but great releasing exercise (from Kiessling 2021), where you sit down with a sheet of paper (folded into four squares or labeled as such). Colored pencils, crayons, or markers are provided to the client for drawing the symptom or trigger. This is an excellent tool to use with younger clients, teens, activated adults, and in a group setting to show how to release intense feelings and emotions.

Steps for Scribble It Out—Four Square
This is adapted from Ignacio "Nacho" Jarero (Kiessling 2021):

1. Divide a piece of paper into four quadrants.

2. Access and activate: Start in the upper left quadrant and ask: "What image, word, or phrase represents the incident? (Actual or abstract, it could be represented by the color of a crayon.) Have the client draw this in the first square.

3. Processing:

   - Ask the client to pick another color crayon/marker, one that may represent a desired, positive, adaptive perspective of the situation.

   - Ask the client to look at the drawing and scribble it out (dual attention stimulation, DAS) using the other color crayon/marker (5–10 seconds) (they may also have tappers in their pockets while scribbling).

   - For the second quadrant, ask the client to notice what has changed or occurred as they think about the incident now, and if a color crayon/marker was used, see if the same one still fits, or if they would like another color. They draw the image, word, or phrase in this second square. Then they scribble it out using what would be the colored crayon/marker that represents how they feel now (DAS, 5–10 seconds while scribbling).

   - Ask the client to continue drawing and scribbling using the remaining squares (front and back if needed) until the drawing or intensity no longer changes.

4. Positive, adaptive strengthening:

   - In one of the remaining blank squares, ask the client to draw how the incident feels now (image, word, phrase), then strengthen those positive thoughts, feelings, and sensations with slow, rhythmic tapping or walking through, i.e., moving their heels up and down as though walking in place (10–15 seconds of stimulation).

5. Integration—draw a future template (optional):

   - In another vacant quadrant, ask the client to draw a future incident related to the original and how it will be adaptively handled, then strengthen those positive thoughts, feelings, and sensations with slow, rhythmic tapping or "walking through," i.e., moving their heels up and down as though walking in place (10–15 seconds of stimulation).

Note: The person may close their eyes in order to have a more vivid image of the positive scenario as it unfolds.

Here is an example of this exercise in action. I used it with a 10-year-old boy who was upset as he was told he could not go on a school trip because of his conduct in school and his grades.

SCRIBBLING OUT ANGER AND DISAPPOINTMENT: THE POWER OF THE CRAYON

In the first square, I asked the boy to describe how he was feeling about not being able to go on the trip (I had him put the pulsing tappers in his pockets while we did this). He said he felt sad (he chose the feeling from a sheet I showed him of faces and feelings), so I had him pick a colored pen and write the word "sad"—and then he scribbled out "sad." Then in the next square, I asked him to describe what he was feeling now about not going on the school trip. He said "mad," so he picked another pen, and wrote down "mad," and scribbled it out. Then he said in the third square he felt overwhelmed. And he picked another pen, wrote that feeling down, and scribbled it out. When I asked him what he was feeling now about going, he said, "Well my mom told me we can go on a trip of our own to New York City." And when he was asked about how he felt about going to New York City with his mom, he said, "Excited, happy, we can do what we want." As he wrote those words down, he also picked out the word "confident" on the list of feelings, so he wrote that down too (I slowed the tappers down while he was writing these).

I asked him if he wanted to scribble these out or keep them. His face lit up and he said "No, I want to focus on New York City now." So, we ended the session with Butterfly Hug and tapped it in around his heart and on his thighs as he said his legs feel happy about this trip. Then we brought his father into the session (who was in the waiting room) to remind him how happy, excited, and confident he felt about his future plans, and how they could both tap it in to remind them of this.

If a client does this exercise outside of the therapy session, they can put it away in their journal, share it with a therapist, or burn it! Just let it go!

A REVISED WAY TO USE SCRIBBLE IT OUT[2]

While I was on an R&R personal retreat at Kripalu Center in Lenox, Massachusetts, (to work on this book and take a workshop with renowned yoga teacher Seane Corn (2019), I took an expressive art class with Dr. Laura Thompson, which, to my surprise and unknown to her (until we talked about it), turned into a variation of Scribble It Out. She gave us all colored pencils and paper and guided us with these instructions:

1. What would you like to let go of? Draw that and scribble it out. We are not free when there is fear, anger, or anxiety present.

2. What obstacles are there? Scribble that out with another colored pencil.

3. Now pick another pencil. What support do you need? What letter do you see in these scribbles? Turn the letter into a word that says something positive about you.

4. Now complete this sentence using that word: I am . . . .

What I saw was the letter "B" and came up with "I am bold" and "I am brave" (to write this book), and "I am beautiful." I added the EMDR piece to it...how true do these feel to me right now (VoC) on a scale of 1–7 where 1 is totally false and 7 is totally true? And how can I strengthen this with an image/sensation, and where do I feel this in my body?... And then I used Butterfly Hug to tap that in.

Feel free to use this when setting an intention, challenging beliefs, and when needed to affirm yourself and feel more confident. Like I did with this exercise, make it yours.

More trauma self-care interventions

As trauma-sensitive clinicians, it is important that we are aware of what we are feeling (the depth of the feelings or sensations in the body) during and after a session. We may even need to notice whether something about our own personal history or family dynamics got activated while working with certain clients or processing incidents. This is when obtaining case consultation, supervision, therapy, and practicing our own self-care is *very important*. In my opinion, this is part of our responsibility in being great trauma-informed clinicians—and falling and staying awake.

It is essential that we recognize and pay attention to how our "stuff" has somehow come into our conscious awareness during our work with clients. When it does, we need to remember to put our stuff on "the shelf," so we can focus on what is going on with our clients. Then later, when working with someone we trust, we can explore: "What came up for me during this session was..." or "What I experienced was..." and examine how our old programming may be trying to get in the way of welcoming new experiences for our clients. As Deb Antinori, Brainspotting expert and lead trainer

---

2   Revised with permission from Dr. Laura Thompson, www.breathingspace.art

said (direct communication, 2023): "We are all human beings and have a nervous system which will be triggered when interacting with others, our clients. How we *respond, recognize, and handle it is so important.* This is the beauty of attunement."

When we are worked up, worried, or not sure what to do for a client, first and foremost, we go for some case consultation. This is to protect our energy and prevent taking on someone else's drama, trauma, or intense situations. Below are several practices you can do to conserve or "protect" your energy.

BECOME AN ASTRONAUT: PUT ON YOUR PROTECTIVE SPACE SUIT

Imagine you are an astronaut and put on your space suit. Put the glass globe head piece over your head and make sure the oxygen is on—wear this imaginary suit (make sure it is zipped up) to protect you from taking on someone else's energy. Feel the negative energy bounce off your head piece and suit, knowing you are protected.

Don't forget to take off the space suit and hang it up in the closet when the session is over, or you no longer feel you need the protection.

SILENCING THE ALARM

If you need to calm yourself or your client down, try this exercise, developed from Donna Eden's work (2008) and taught by Robin Shapiro (personal communication, 2023) and available on YouTube.[3] Here is the script:

> Close your eyes and think of what is troubling or upsetting you. As you inhale, cross at the wrists and bring opposite hands up to the eyebrow center. As you start to exhale, the fingers (left hand over the right eye, right hand over the left eye) gently start to massage the eyebrows making their way to the sides of the eyes, to the ears massaging the ears, gentle tug at the ear lobes, continuing to exhale as you massage the back of the neck, the shoulders, upper arms, and with a final exhale (arms are crossed in front of the heart at this point) release the arms at the sides with a strong exhale out of the mouth, letting all that was on your mind go.
>
> Do this with your client (or for yourself) three times, and then relax the arms and remain in stillness for a moment, returning to normal slow breathing. Notice what you are sensing now, and, when you are ready, breathe out through the mouth slowly and open your eyes. How do you feel?

---

3   www.youtube.com/watch?v=R-oshgfe2SE

SILENCING THE ALARM: CASE EXAMPLE FROM AN EMDR THERAPIST

I was scheduled for EMDR consultation group on a recent Friday. I had several highly distressing and stressful things going on in my personal life. I almost cancelled but showed up as I felt it would not be right cancelling last minute. I was distracted, unsettled, could feel my gut churning and my heart pounding. I shared some of what was going on with my group and was clearly distressed while doing so. Dr. Kathy asked if we could try a technique called Silencing the Alarm and I/the other group members agreed. I was skeptical that my alarm could be silenced. I was shocked when, after two times of doing this, my gut had settled, my heart felt normal, and I actually felt calm. I could hardly believe it had worked so quickly. I've had the opportunity to share this with several of my therapy clients as well as with patients at the hospital where I work. Each person has reported the same kind of instant calming. I absolutely *love this tool*!!

COMPLICATED GRIEF: CASE EXAMPLE

Sometimes we have to modify, adapt, and try other things. Shay is a 73-year-old female who sought out therapy four years ago, "feeling stuck" after losing her wife to a long and complicated illness. They were married for 29 years.

This is what she said about EMDR: "I don't really understand EMDR. Thoughts may come into my mind, and you say, 'Okay, go with that.' When these sessions are over, I usually feel disoriented and confused and I don't know why. I have never felt calm, enlightened, or felt that I benefited from this."

And about Brainspotting: "I don't like this at all. Staring at one point for a length of time is difficult. Even finding the 'spot' to look was challenging. I found this exhausting, and I felt confused and disoriented at the end of every session when we did this. It never seemed to help me."

When we used Yoga Nidra and EMDR together, this was her response:

Twice I have attended Yoga Nidra and have done EMDR in the same day. This seemed to open my mind somewhat and I don't feel as "stuck." Both times I have had energy and motivation to accomplish things in my business and my personal life and felt productive and good about it. My mind seems to "clear up" when these are done together as it seems to open up the logjam in my head. It removes the conflict of doing something or just avoiding doing anything such as going out and enjoying the outside. I think EMDR pinpoints where the logjam is in my mind and the Yoga Nidra disperses it. I wonder what would happen if I had Yoga Nidra and EMDR back-to-back several times? I wonder if the energy and motivation would last longer?

After she shared this with me, we decided we were going to try this and "Go with that!"

Triggers/symptoms—more about what they are telling you

If you have read this far, you are beginning to fall awake, creating a different relationship with and respect for your brain, the physical body, and the science associated with symptoms, aches, diagnosis, beliefs, and repeated patterns of behavior. This perspective provides the space to focus on the meaning and message of these and discover what you can do to intervene on your behalf. Conventional Western medicine advocates handling a symptom by getting rid of it as fast as possible, such as just taking medication—and the more uncomfortable the symptom is, the bigger the dose is often prescribed to obliterate it. Although we need to acknowledge and value the major contributions of medical science and modern medicine, there is much more we can be proactive about in our activities of daily living, including following a doctor's orders.

Until we listen to the message of the symptom and what our mind and body is trying to tell us (the headache, back pain, immune disorder, tight hips, lack of sleep, asthma, cancer), the body will continue to exacerbate symptoms in one form or another, such as a physical emergency, acting as an additional alarm (in addition to the brain) "forcing us to pay attention." If you hold a belief that physical symptoms have no meaning besides your bodily discomfort, deserving the attention of only a physician, I suggest you suspend this way of thinking and be curious about learning more about your anatomy and physiology. Your Committee (remember them?) will be more than glad to hold onto to this way of suffering until you decide to pay attention to it, inquire about behavior, and perhaps heal yourself.

Diana Spiess, MS, has created a community of health and wellness education at her Yoga and Pilates Studio in Maumee, Ohio. In her relaxation classes, she integrates movement, sound, and intention, emphasizing that everything we think, eat, and do, and how we socialize, impacts our wellness. Having a community of healing is also very important. This place provided me a place of refuge and support while I was in Ohio during my mom's health decline and death.

CALM/COMFORTABLE/PEACEFUL PLACE EXERCISE

EMDR, Brainspotting, and Yoga Nidra also use grounding techniques, known as mental imagery or cueing to sensation. These grounding exercises help diffuse the intensity of emotions, feelings, and thoughts being experienced in the moment. What is also important to remember is that people find some grounding exercises more helpful than others. That is why it is suggested you look at several of those outlined here, or perhaps one of your own, to use on yourself or with clients. They all utilize the five senses to disrupt or create space from the intense thoughts, triggers, stressors, and feelings. This is to distract the left brain from "looping" or going back into the analytical thinking mind.

While there are many grounding exercises, another one that can easily be integrated into your practice is visual grounding called mental imagery (everybody has an imagination). This one invites the client to imagine a calm, comfortable place that they have either been to before or seen in a movie or magazine that looks like a place where they can feel calm, secure, and at ease. And if nothing comes to mind, they can just see the word "peace" or the word "calm" in their mind's eye. Often, intense thoughts lead to feeling unsafe. With this grounding technique, you can feel and access calming sensations while also distracting yourself from those thoughts and intense feelings that are real but not true now (remember how stories get created).

Here is another exercise that you can do anywhere and anytime (with tapping and Butterfly Hug, if you like, to reinforce the neural networks, with the intention to relax and be calm):

1. Sit down and place your feet on the ground, hands separated (not touching) on the thighs, palms facing up.

2. Allow yourself to land where you are and acknowledge the time you are taking for you.

3. Slowly, take deep breaths out and shorter inhales through the nose.

4. Close your eyes partially or fully, or even keep them open—focusing on something soothing—whatever feels more comfortable.

5. Now think of a place that you like and that makes you feel calm, comfortable, at ease —real or imagined, it does not matter.

6. Start with a visual image of the place, what it looks like. Focus on and notice the details about the place.

7. Hear the sounds, smells, or temperature the place has.

8. Notice any and all physical sensations of this place—for example, the sand on the beach, the wind, trees, or maybe a blanket under or over you.

9. As you're visualizing, notice and feel any comforting emotions you're feeling, like happiness, coziness, or calm.

10. Think of a phrase that represents the visual image and say it to yourself.

11. If you like you can slowly tap this in place or combine it with Butterfly Hug. And when you are ready, breathe out through your mouth slowly and open your eyes. Notice what you are feeling now.

As you work with clients and use the brain therapies, here are a few concepts to remember as a session unfolds (de Shazer and Dolan 2007):

- If it isn't broken, don't fix it ("stay in the tail of the comet;" see Chapter 4).

- If it works, do more of it ("go from there").

- If it's not working, do something different ("stay curious").

- Small steps can lead to big changes ("take baby steps").

- The solution is not necessarily directly related to the problem ("we don't have to know why it works other than it does").

- The language for solution development is different from that needed to describe a problem ("words have power"; see Shafer 2010).

- No problem happens all the time; there are always exceptions that can be utilized ("draw on memories of success").

- The future is both created and negotiable ("making what seems impossible possible").

If helpful, they can refer to these if they are activated between sessions and need to calm down.

Now that you are learning that brainbody therapies are event-driven (something brought them to you), belief-based (the nervous system is out of balance based on stories), a memory about something has been activated/resurfaced and is upsetting (need to find the source or part from the past that is activated), you have tools to regulate and remain calm. There are many ways to "see" the situation and what actions to take. What is resonating with you now? *Imagine* what you can do and keep *falling awake. Here, shift happens.*

CHAPTER 8

Now What? On-Demand Tools for Falling and Remaining Awake

In this chapter, you start thinking about how you can integrate a falling awake plan for you and your clients. You are now in charge of your own self-regulation and how it works. The brainbody therapies are a neurological system regulator that heals from the bottom up/top down, left/right whole brain healing at the same time (Chapter 2). This "drama no more" (DNM) is a comprehensive life management approach for falling awake—using The FUN® Program as a stand-alone practice or integrating it with the brain therapies of EMDR, Brainspotting, and/or Yoga Nidra. What is suggested is that you create a plan that's flexible and right for *you*, which may vary and change depending on what is going on for you now and in the future.

At this point, I think you are aware that the first step in designing your lifestyle management plan is that you assume responsibility for creating it, implementing it daily, and believing that you are your own best primary care provider. And when you need help implementing this or some guidance of what to do, seek out a trained therapist or take a workshop or training that specializes in the brainbody therapies mentioned here.

When we embrace the uncertainty principle, nothing happens by chance

While working on this chapter, I found the journal in which I wrote down all the mental imagery exercises and teachings I learned from Dr. Gerald Epstein's teacher, Colette Aboulker-Muscat, who lived in Jerusalem (I went there three times to learn from her). After landing in Tel Aviv, I would ask the taxi driver to take me to the house with the blue gate in Jerusalem (I was by myself; Dr. Epstein told me Colette did not have an address and to tell the cab driver those instructions). Interestingly enough, my journal is dated June 9, 1994, which was around three months before I was hit by a car and wrote The FUN® Program. I also worked on this chapter the day war broke out again in Israel (October 7, 2023). Using the power of mental imagery that Dr. Epstein and Colette taught me, let's stop here for a moment, close our eyes, exhale slowly three times, and imagine and see world peace... Think about the lyrics to "Imagine" by John Lennon... And pause...

The following incorporates some of the teachings from Colette that I have implemented in my work over the past 30 years for falling and remaining awake.

The keys to implementing The FUN® Program, and any of the brain therapies, include checking on the activities of the Committee and remembering the benefits that can be gained by *not talking* or *thinking* (implement the WAIT acronym: What Am I Thinking? Why Am I Thinking? Why Am I Talking?). According to Colette, taking risks in the physical world, which is leaping into uncertainty (that Brainspotting word again), is movement toward getting what you want (Chapter 2, First Session Exercise). Taking risks embraces life, which is breaking the habits of who you thought you were and becoming all you are meant to be. (Whew! Thanks Colette!)

To review, while each of the brainbody therapies can be used in diverse situations and for a variety of reasons, here is what they all have in common:

1. Selecting an event to process and putting pressure on the neural networks by use of eye movements (BLS)/brainspot/eyes open or closed, mental imagery, alternating tones through bilateral music, or alternating tactile stimulation (tapping, movement). These all acknowledge cortical activity while simultaneously creating a vividness and intensity of emotions, eventually helping the brainbody self-regulate and share insights gained.

2. Each therapy is providing healing by what is called bottom-up processing (from the limbic "basement brain" to the prefrontal cortex, the "upstairs brain"). The eye movements and mental imagery modulate brainwave frequencies (high and slow brainwave frequencies), providing hippocampus access and cortical integration (see Chapter 1). Depending on what was discovered, a neurological switch is flipped, making shifts happen, processing information from implicit memory networks to explicit memory networks, and from episodic to semantic memory networks, enabling the calmer cortical brain to think about what we want to say or do (movement from the "History" to the "Discovery" channel).

3. Orienting and focusing on an incident without the actual danger/disturbance/trauma present (sympathetic nervous system activation) during the treatment session allows for the ventral vagal circuit to turn on (parasympathetic nervous system). This potentially enables access to consolidation (making sense) of disturbing experiences without avoiding them (e.g., "No wonder I felt that way or created that belief about myself"). This allows space for alternating between reexperiencing and reflecting.

4. The therapies put pressure on the working memory via dual attention stimulation, focusing simultaneously on several processes at the same time (the incident and the stimulation, thought, or sensation); for example, the ability to feel calm although upset, able to release upset, and also interested about

alternatives. Putting pressure on the neural networks while focusing on the stimulation or sensation wears on the working memory, reducing its vividness and emotionality. This creates psychological distance from the memory and behavioral response. Simply saying, "What do you notice now?" or "go from there," or actually being in deeper states of consciousness (Yoga Nidra), allows the adaptive information processing (AIP) system to experience from and observe witnessing self-reflection to keep what is important and to discard what is no longer helpful (emotions and beliefs).

In all these approaches, healing occurs first when the there is a caring, regulated, attuned, attentive, secure, consistent relationship that is established between the client and the provider. Regardless of the portal clients enter for help (how they find us), all clients will expand their window of tolerance and learn self-regulation tools to use in their daily life for integration. Clients also learn that during processing (in session), other developmental stages of information may be accessed that were not obtainable or realized in other talk therapies.

Please know that it takes time for "transformation"—remember, it can take 21 days to change or create a new habit or change in behavior or beliefs. While miracles can and do happen (yes, single session therapy is possible), know that the process of change usually takes time and dedication. Also know that you or your clients will go off track at times or find yourself in relapse or reactive mode. This is why lifestyle management programs are flexible and kind and can always be adjusted to begin again. In my first book, I referred to a poem called "Autobiography in Five Chapters" that sheds light on this process (Shafer and Greenfield 2000, p.79):

- Chapter One: I walk down the street. There's a deep hole in the sidewalk. I fall in, I am lost. I am hopeless. It isn't my fault. It takes me forever to find a way out.

- Chapter Two: I walk down the same street. There is a deep hole in the sidewalk. I pretend I don't see it. I fall in again. I can't believe I'm in the same place. But it isn't my fault. It still takes a long time to get out.

- Chapter Three: I walk down the same street. There's a deep hole in the sidewalk. I see it is there. I still fall in—it is a habit. My eyes are open, I know where I am. It is my fault. I get out immediately.

- Chapter Four: I walk down the same street. There is a deep hole in the sidewalk. I walk around it.

- Chapter Five: I walk down another street...

Finally! How many of us can relate to this process of going down the same street?! Several times, or we keep hitting the repeat button? With this in mind—since we are now *falling and hope to remain awake*...how about trying this for starters:

Implement The FUN® Program for falling awake with the AAA plan: Awake,

Attuned, Aware. Now you may be asking, but which program or type of processing is the "one"—for you and/or your clients? It is not about which method, what app, the protocol, or script, but about designing your own recovery and self-care. Part of that includes having a tribe (your team). Some examples of tribe connections are: the Inner Resource System (IRS); a yoga or exercise community; a 12-step recovery program; individual and/or group therapy; meeting with a shaman; joining a church, temple, meditation group; or going on a retreat. In other words, go outside, find your inner and outer tribe, and connect with yourself and others.

Here are some guidelines that may help you decide which program to start with or suggest:

- The FUN® Program for the anxious, driven, results-oriented, need-to-talk, cortical folks (no judgment).

- EMDR for complex situations; for folks who don't want to or need to talk, who are not sure where to start, or who specifically say, "I want EMDR" because they heard about it.

- Brainspotting for folks who tried talk therapy and EMDR and either those therapies did not work or they didn't "like" them, "nothing happened," or they did not have a good connection to the therapist/healing practitioner, and/or still do not want to do much talking or talk about the past.

- Yoga Nidra for folks who don't trust therapists or yogis ("yoga is a cult") and who don't want to talk or move—but claim they are stressed. They can just show up, sit or lie down, and see what happens—no movement or talking or sharing required.

First, remember that you are working with a *person* and not an issue or a diagnosis. No matter what "technique," advanced protocol, EMDR, Brainspotting, or Yoga Nidra "script," sound bowls you are hearing, gemstones you are touching, or other bells and whistles you bring into the healing session, remember that you and your client are the "expert" on what you need or where "feels" right to begin. What you and your client are connecting to is the relationship between you. Recovery is about connection. There is a short, animated video on YouTube called Rat Park[1] that explains quickly why some people get addicted to drugs and others don't—depending on *relationships*. Think of all this as taking your remote and switching from the "History" to the "Discovery" channel...or maybe even the "Travel" channel once the imagination gets involved.

---

1   www.youtube.com/watch?v=xNmEboNEnd8

The stigma of seeking help or support

> *The world we have created is a product of our thinking; it cannot be changed without changing our thinking. (Albert Einstein)*

Unfortunately, asking for or seeking help still carries stigma, implying that the person is weak or mentally ill, or it invites the Committee and the Monkey Mind to start chatting and jumping. For example, even therapists may be ashamed or not admit that they need or are seeking help (even if it is to take time for themselves given how much they give to others). I believe that the best approach is to not ask others if you should try therapy. If your "gut" is telling you to do it, trust your own inner expert/Authority.

We live in a society where millions of people have been impacted by trauma, illness, addiction, mental illness, accidents, man-made disasters, or acts of nature (fires, floods, tornados, hurricanes, blizzards, etc.). These events impact everybody differently, and access to mental health services (lack of or no insurance coverage) for many professionals specifically trained in the brainbody therapies may be an out-of-pocket expense and you will hear, "You charge what?" or "I can't afford that; I'll just talk to a friend." Stigma, shaming, and embarrassing situations affect all of us—and nearly everyone has felt stigmatized or has judged others at some point in their lives, due to racism, generational trauma, lack of education, culture, or beliefs held about what happened to them. When it comes to mental health and addiction treatment, there is a profound lack of access and adherence (staying committed to the process), either due to the shame in asking for it or the inability to access or afford it, not knowing where to turn for the level of care needed, or the therapy is "not working fast enough"—"you are not fixing what I came for."

Seeking professional help happens to all of us, whether it is a dentist, physical therapist, hairdresser, mental health professional, physician, or a psychiatrist (notice how you felt in your brainbody about admitting to seeing some of these, especially those on the end of the list). We can all do a better job of decreasing stigma and increasing access for mental health and substance misuse treatment, embracing the concepts mentioned in Chapter 1 of kindness, compassion, and consideration, understanding that everybody has a lot going on (we never know unless it is made known).

The refusal or stigma that can negatively impact someone (or ourselves) asking for or seeking help, can include:

- Our willingness to talk to "a stranger" (e.g., "I can talk to a friend").

- Our difficulty making mental healthcare accessible or inclusive (e.g., "I don't have insurance," "The person I want to see doesn't accept insurance, and I'll end up being out of pocket if I pay").

- Keeping things secret (e.g., "I have kept it all private for so long, what's the point of talking about it now?").

- Self-esteem (e.g., "Other people have worse things going on than I do;" "What must I believe about myself to deny (or devalue) my own needs this way?") (Maté 2022. p.418).

- Questioning our mental health (e.g., "People who go to therapy are "f***ed up." If that is the case, then I am because I go!").

STIGMA CASE EXAMPLE

Johnny, who we met in the EMDR chapter, is a 54-year-old married male referred for PTSD. He was a New York City police officer who moved to Florida. He was referred to me by his psychiatrist for mood stabilization and anger management. Johnny felt like the psychiatrist was over-medicating him and was not interested in treating him. He had had a stroke and was frustrated because since it did not occur while he was on duty as a police officer, he was still required to report back to duty as a law enforcement officer. He disclosed to me that "being a cop you are not allowed to have feelings—if they find out you are in therapy, they will strip you of your badge as you are deemed 'unable' to perform your duties, hence the high rate of suicide in the police department."

Johnny shared that his breakthrough in therapy was when I introduced him to EMDR and told him to hold the tappers and to put everything else that came up into the container. He continues to remind me to this day that the container exercise, tappers, and learning how to relax and breathe saved his life. "I haven't lashed out at anyone since. While there is no 'cure,' therapy is my medication—not what was being prescribed to me by the psychiatrist. It took me a couple of years in therapy to be able to function again in society."

The impact of stigma on treatment

Unfortunately, people who experience stigma about their inability to "fix it themselves" are less likely to seek treatment—and this results in economic, social, and increased medical costs. In the United States in 2000, costs associated with untreated addiction (including those related to healthcare, criminal justice, and lost productivity) amounted to a whopping $510 billion (Miller and Hendrie 2008)—imagine what that cost is now!

Perceived stigma in hospitals, by doctors, or in the psychotherapy office can discourage people from accessing behavioral health services. Having a trusted primary care doctor is associated with maintaining well-being and a good quality of life (we know this is hard to find as our current medical system is broken—unless you can afford the luxury lifestyle management known as "concierge services"). However, some studies have found that some healthcare providers often feel uncomfortable when working with people who have behavioral health issues, mood disturbances, or are misusing alcohol and drugs (Brondani, Alan, and Donnelly 2017). In a study of attitudes towards these presenting issues, the majority of healthcare professionals held negative views about people who misuse alcohol or drugs, or failed to look at physical and emotional problems that may be due to lifestyle choices (poor diet, loneliness, addiction, lack of exercise or hobbies, etc.) (Beltrán-Carrillo *et al.* 2022).

The bias a provider (embracing a stigma) can have working with clients presenting with these problems can influence patient outcomes. Individuals who feel they are "just a number," being seen for only 10 minutes, whose phone calls are not returned (even by the referring clinician) may choose not to seek help altogether. According to Maté (2022, p.242): "...diagnoses reveal nothing about the *underlying events and dynamics that animate the perceptions and experiences in question*. They keep our gaze trained on effects and not the myriad of their causes" (emphasis added). These can include domestic and sexual violence, poverty, substance misuse, immune disorders, the death of a pet, a complicated divorce, or being bullied at work or in grade school.

These events that happen in a toxic culture or family dysfunction can lead to the person (or ourselves) feeling ashamed or embarrassed, believing "I will never get better," "I'm a loser," "I never want to ask for help," or "If this gets out, I'm screwed."

Finally seeking treatment

When considering the course of treatment or which professional to see, here are some things to ponder:

- Starting the self-care/recovery journey is a huge first step. Remember, you and your clients are the ones ready to start doing something different (Nelson 2010). Unfortunately, those who may need it most may never dare to take such a courageous leap (those who think everyone else is the problem or the one "to blame" are the ones who really should go). Usually, the people seeking help are talking about the people or family members who won't go.

- The work/research you do up front is investing in your healthcare. Check out several therapists and ask a lot of questions. Ask about their credentials and make sure they are real.

- Remember that everyone can benefit from therapy. It's like going to a gym— you have to use and like the equipment that is being recommended.

- Treat yourself with nice cream—seeking help from a professional is a sign of strength, not weakness. Remember, it is your choice (unless you are being mandated for some reason such as an intervention, arrest, or illness—and even then, you still have choices).

- Be open and curious about different methods and specialties. Ask the professionals you are considering about their training and where they received it. Ask how long they have been practicing.

- Ask if they offer in-person sessions and/or have telehealth options.

- Find out exactly what your insurance providers pay so you are not surprised about reimbursement rates. Don't let insurance companies tell you they pay 100 percent—they do not. They pay 100 percent of what they decide their contracted rate is. If you are paying out of pocket, ask the provider if they have a sliding fee scale.

- Ask if they provide group therapy, workshops, or other classes where you can learn more about the therapy they provide.

- Don't get discouraged if it takes a while to find the right "fit" or "connection." Sharing your private world with someone is a very personal and private matter, and this provider must feel comfortable (yes, we are all eager to stand in line outside a therapy office, waiting for our turn to talk to someone about things that are upsetting us) and welcoming to you.

- All your questions are important—please ask them. Remember, all healthcare providers are people too. And remember that sometimes therapists have bad days too (they may have to cancel, be running late, have to leave town, have a family or unexpected emergency, or get sick). But if things seem to keep happening and it is not working, seek help elsewhere.

Here are some of the questions I sometimes get asked when I first meet people, or during the course of my work or interaction with them on the phone, in my office, or on Zoom:

- Do you care about your clients?

- Do you feel a connection between us?

- Do you think I am getting better?

- Do you think you can help me?

- What are you going to do or recommend for me? I need a plan.

- Have you worked with someone like me before (adoption, addiction, bipolar, sex offender, domestic violence, LBGTQ+, straight, Black, White, Hispanic, My Tribe, etc.)? Notice how people describe themselves. I often say back: "Have you ever worked with someone like me before (therapist, White female)? If so, was it helpful?" Or what would they like to know about me?

In the four decades I have been in private practice, I have been asked and challenged by many things and questions, and for me the most important thing is to be authentic and real. When I don't know or am not sure, I say it, or I may ask my client how they feel about what they are asking me...what would they like me to know? I may also let them know I will look into something I don't have an answer for at that moment, or if I am not the best trained professional in this modality or for this issue, I may offer to find someone (but this is also challenging, as referral sources may not be a good fit either).

The practitioner as guide

Some trauma-informed providers consider Yoga Nidra, EMDR, and Brainspotting as integrative, somatic, neuroexperiential, and a mindbody form of personal transformation. As we have seen in this book, when these therapies are used, the brain lights up and strengthens those neural pathways that are ready to access areas in the memory network for healing (neurons that fire together wire together). Setting an intention or focus for the session jolts the system out of the default mode network (DMN) and ignites an innate energetic process and curiosity of self-inquiry that is not accessed by traditional talk therapies. This brings awareness to intense emotions, stories, or beliefs, separating us from ourselves and the world around you (where attention goes, energy flows).

Using these approaches for healing-suppressed, stuck, or ruminating thinking, the role of the practitioner is that of a guide. Not much discussion or dialogue is needed other than to encourage the client to go in, "notice that," or "go from there," or "that sounds important." Kaelen (2017) proposes an extended view of the snow globe metaphor from Chapter 1, viewing the brain in this way:

> Think of the brain as a hill covered in snow, and thoughts as sleds gliding down that hill. As one sled after another goes down the hill, a small number of main trails will appear in the snow. And every time a new sled goes down, it will be drawn into the preexisting trails, almost like a magnet.

This represents how the DMN becomes stronger and stronger, making it seem impossible to consider any other path or direction. When the worn-down brain forest trails appear, the steady, regulated, attuned therapist holds the intention/belief/target/issue, so that the person can slow down, pause, process, and then continue. When the client continues, they can go in other directions, explore new landscapes, and literally create new pathways or find their way back to the original path to process some more. When the path is freshest, the mind is most impressionable, and the slightest movement or nudge, whether a sound or suggestion from the therapist, can powerfully influence the course of the therapy session (Pollan 2018).

At the end of the session, the client and therapist usually attain a sense of relief and peace in the brainbody in the present moment (now you/the client have some new tools to try to keep this going). Since all the healing modalities and approaches in this book can be offered in-person, by Zoom, or as on-demand practices, they can be accessed and practiced anytime, anywhere. Therefore, support on how to respond mindfully to life experiences is always available—no matter what is going on in it *now*.

The following three factors may also assist you when considering which approach may be more appropriate for you and your client:

- The trauma history is not extensive; it is an isolated event. These situations are less challenging (sometimes) to work with than multiple complex traumas, which may need to be approached in parts.

- The ability to work through and overcome the issue is positively influenced when the client has a kind, supportive, caring support system (referring again to that animated Rat Park video on YouTube). If the client is surrounded by a tribe (e.g., family members, a coach, an employer) who continue to react to them with impatience, criticism, or humiliation, this continued emotional abuse further traumatizes them, impacting the likelihood of success, and can complicate the treatment process. The therapist may need to discuss this with the client and help them find a supportive tribe.

- Helping an individual work through complex emotions, fears, and attachments is more complicated if the individual is clinically depressed, has an anxiety disorder, or is active in an addiction. This calls for more case conceptualization and resource development, which is possible but more complicated and time consuming. Always resort back to your clinical or case management skills or seek out consultation to help you with your decision-making and treatment planning.

Therapy rooted in the neural-biophysiological responses of the body offers opportunities for deep self-inquiry that go beyond traditional talk therapy (refer back to the acronym WAIT: Why Am I Talking?/What Am I Thinking? Or WAIST: Why Am I Still Talking?). The human body is an intricately wired connective tissue system of thoughts, emotions, and physical reactions. What happens in one system affects all the others. This dynamic is one reason behind the effectiveness of these brainbody approaches.

Think of *The Wizard of Oz*. At first, Dorothy's world was very simple and black and white—it was just her, Auntie Em, and Toto. Then the cyclone showed up, disrupted her world, and carried her off into another world—literally. When she landed, she opened the door to find herself in a place she had never seen before, and it was full of color and new people who were strangers to her. Just like Dorothy on the yellow brick road, the more we delve in and explore ourselves and our healing through these brain-based therapies, the more we get curious and want to learn more about them. Through them, we and our clients will learn that, like Dorothy, we have had the power all along to be in charge of our own thoughts and behavior.

This is what happens when we fall awake, challenge our thoughts and beliefs, and try something *different*. Here are some resourcing exercises for you to try.

These on-demand tools are excellent options to use in response to stress, feeling stuck, or needing a "time out" or some calm—in the therapy session or out in the world. They can also be beneficial for attending to sensations and symptoms. Simply, the intensity of a sensation or emotion is allowing the brainbody space to speak on its own terms, without trying to analyze and without drawing conclusions or making up stories about it. Its voice might be heard during a mental imagery exercise, while writing in a journal, during a dream, or as part of a spontaneous insight that seems to come out of "nowhere."

GO OUTSIDE AND FIND A TREE

Lean against a tree and look up—notice something beautiful. Know that the tree has your back and won't let you down. Once you do this exercise, you will always be looking for that tree that is singing to you "lean on me" (like the Bill Withers song).

BUTTERFLY HUG (ALSO KNOWN AS ANGEL WINGS AND HEART HUG, AND TAPPING IT IN)

The originator of Butterfly Hug, according to Dr. Ignacio ("Nacho) Jarero (2023), is Lucina Artigas. In February 1998, an EMDR team was invited to assist Hurricane Paulina's survivors in Acapulco, Mexico. Jarero, an internationally renowned EMDR clinician and trainer, was the team leader who asked Artigas to conduct the closure exercise. She was playing with a four-year-old boy who, between laughs, asked her: "And when you return home, who will hug me?" Artigas put herself in the center of the team and, spontaneously inspired by this, closed the event with what is now known as Butterfly Hug. This example demonstrates the mindful and creative way Butterfly Hug can be used with diverse populations and settings. Butterfly Hug can also be used as an exercise to help with setting an intention for Yoga Nidra, and/or to close down an EMDR or Brainspotting session to "tap in" what the client reports they found helpful or calming while processing.

As you have been reading, bilateral stimulation (BLS), also known as "tapping," can be immensely helpful when revisiting or working through traumatic, stressful experiences or when triggered to engage in self-harm (drugs, alcohol, violence, cutting, gambling, etc.). Many situations in life can bring back our "stuff"—such as intense emotions or memories, feeling like the past is present again—causing distress.

If this occurs and you are triggered, you can self-administer one of the resource-tapping methods (also used in Thought Field Therapy and Emotional Freedom Techniques founded in the 1990s by Dr. Roger Callahan and Gary Craig) and tapping it in during EMDR (Parnell 2008, 2018; see also Kase 2023; Knipe 2009; Shapiro 2016). The tapping and BLS method is popular in some talk therapies and EMDR, and used while focusing on the distress or resource while engaging in tactile stimulation (tapping). While it's part of the grounding or processing techniques used in these therapies, you can also use it on its own as an exercise during distressing or anxious situations to calm yourself (silencing the alarm center of the amygdala) and bring yourself to the present.

1. Cross your arms over your chest and interlock your thumbs (forming a butterfly) so that your middle fingers are right below the collar bone or clavicle and the

remaining fingers touch the K26 spot, the soft notch below the collarbone, which is energetically soothing. Other forms of Butterfly Hug have the arms crossed with the hands placed on the shoulders or arms. If you want you can lock the hands in place by hooking in the thumbs at the heart center (this is optional, and not done if you are placing the hands on the shoulders or arms). Choose the hand position of your choice.

2. Make sure each hand touching the opposite side of the heart, shoulders, and elbows is relaxed (or on opposite shoulders/arms).

3. Close your eyes or soften the gaze.

4. Now move the hands, alternating them one at a time as if you're imitating the movement of butterfly wings.

5. While you are slowly moving your hands bilaterally, make sure to focus on your breath, with long, slow exhales.

6. Observe what is going through your mind, perhaps the upsetting situation, thoughts, and emotions.

7. Allow and welcome all thoughts, feelings, and sensations; just notice them. They are visitors, members of the Committee coming to give you information.

8. If you like, see the thoughts in your mind floating away like moving clouds in the sky, passing by slowly and vanishing from sight, or like leaves flowing down a river or stream. Let them all go. In fact, as you do this, you can inhale the word "let" and exhale the word "go."

9. When you feel ready to come back to the present, taking your time, breathe out through your mouth slowly and open your eyes. Notice what you are sensing now. What has shifted, been released? Be curious about your awareness now.

The intention of this exercise is to welcome all that is arising, thank all thoughts, sensations, and emotions for visiting, understand why they have come, and then let them go.

THE PENDULUM

This is very good for becoming unstuck. Intention: To become unstuck.

1. Breathe in and out three times, short inhales through the nostrils, longer exhales out of the mouth.

2. Imagine you are in front of a pendulum. Put two fingers on either side of the thread of the pendulum. See it swing back and forth, from the right to the left. As it swings to the right, notice it stops at the place where you feel stuck is (your pain, discomfort, disease, etc.).

3. Now see a teaspoon pick up some of the crystals from the right (from this place of pain, discomfort, etc.) within you and swing the pendulum—with the crystals—far to the left, throwing the crystals away, off into the horizon to the left. Continue doing this back and forth—swinging to the right and taking the crystals to the left. Continue this process, and, when the crystals are completely moved from the right to the left, picture the pendulum taking all the crystals further to the left to make a wide flow of stars like the "tail of a comet."

4. See the crystals go up through the clouds and into the universe and beyond into the stratosphere. Pause.

5. Then see a light crystal rain (or heavier) come down from above, purifying you inside and out.*

6. When you are ready, breathe out through your mouth and open your eyes.

*A person can also see the rain come down for a longer period, depending on the severity of the situation or healing need. When the eyes re-open, inquire: "How do you feel?" If the report is a good sensation or experience, tap it in (refer to Butterfly Hug in Chapter 3). If not, or the person remains "stuck" in the "right-hand" issues, explore how to do more variations of the exercise and "go from there."

LIGHT STREAM

With this exercise (Shapiro 2001), the therapist asks the client to bring a disturbing target to mind and to notice the resulting changes in body sensations. The therapist repeats the procedure until the client is easily able to identify body sensations that accompany the disturbing material. Once the client is able to concentrate on the body sensations, the visualization proceeds. The therapist tells the client that this is an imaginal exercise and that there are no right or wrong answers. The therapist then asks the client to concentrate on body sensations:

1. "Concentrate on the feeling in your body. If the feeling had a shape, what would it be?"

2. After the client responds, the therapist continues with, "And if it had a size, what would it be?"

3. The therapist continues this line of questioning by asking about the feeling's color, temperature, texture, and sound (e.g., "If it had a color, what would it be?"). When clients are asked about the feeling's sound, they are told to simply describe it as "high-pitched or low;" otherwise they might become frustrated or anxious by trying to make the sound.

4. After the client has responded to these questions, they are asked, "Which of

your favorite colors might you associate with healing?" It is important that the therapist accept the client's answer—unless it is the same one offered for the color of the feeling in the body. In this case, the therapist should ask for another color.

5. Once the client identifies a color, the therapist continues as follows: "Imagine that this favorite-colored light is coming in through the top of your head and directing itself at the shape in your body. Let's pretend that the source of this light is the cosmos: The more you see, the more you have available. The light directs itself at the shape and penetrates and permeates it, resonating and vibrating in and around it. As it does, what happens to the shape, size, or color?"

6. If the client indicates that it is changing in any way, the therapist continues, repeating a version of the words in the previous step, and asking for feedback until the shape is completely gone, has become transparent, has assumed the same color as the light, or has undergone some other transformation. Change in the image usually correlates with the disappearance of the upsetting feeling.

7. If no change occurs after the second attempt (the client might say, "Nothing is happening; the light is just bouncing off"), the technique should be discontinued and another one tried.

8. After the feeling that accompanies the disturbing material dissipates, the therapist may continue in a slow, soothing tone:

As the light continues to direct itself to that area, you can allow the light to come in and gently and easily fill your entire head. Now, allow it to descend through your neck, into your shoulders, and down your arms into your hands and out your fingertips. Now, allow it to come down your neck and into the trunk of your body, easily and gently. Now, allow it to descend through your buttocks into your legs, streaming down your legs and flowing out your feet.

9. Once the therapist perceives that the client is fully relaxed, the client is given a positive suggestion for peace and calm until the next session.

10. The client is then asked to become fully awake and aware on the count of five.

LIGHT STREAM (VARIATION TO SHUT DOWN AN INCOMPLETE OR INTENSE SESSION)

Here is an outline for this variation (Shafer 2023):

1. "Take a deep breath and let out a long, slow exhale. Please allow your eyes to close or soften your gaze as you enter the world of imagination (everybody has one). Remember, there is no right way or wrong way to do this exercise, only your

way. The intention is to help you feel calm and relaxed as we end the session for today. Are you ready?" (See if you can get a mental nod—if not, you may need another way of shutting down the session or another exercise.)

2. "As you slow your breathing down, bring your attention to the bottom of your feet. As you do this, notice that on the bottom of your feet there is a trap door, and out of the bottom of your feet is flowing a beautiful healing color of light." (Ask them what the color is and the sensation they feel. If it is calming, continue—if not, try something else or ask them what they would like to feel *around* the bottom of the feet and continue.)

3. Tell them that "this beautiful healing color of light is going around the feet and ankles, making its way around the whole body, up the legs, tail bone, front/back/sides of the body, both arms, hands, up to the shoulders, up the neck, relaxing the face, both ears, and the whole head, including the brain. Then there appears another trap door at the top of the head [if that worked with the feet; otherwise, just say around the top of the head] and that healing color of light is now pouring out of the top of the head, down around the whole body, like a cocoon surrounding you with the healing color of light all the way back down to your feet."

4. Pause. Ask them how they feel. If they are calm, tell them to enjoy this sensation and ask if they want to keep this healing energy of light on or put it away for now.

5. When they tell you, ask them to very gently come back into the room when they are ready by breathing out slowly and opening their eyes.

6. Then ask: "How do you feel?" If they report something calm, or good, you can tap it in (Butterfly Hug) and encourage them to practice this calming exercise often. If they say they felt nothing or anxious, consider exploring the Blocking Beliefs Questionnaire at the next session.

VARIATION OF THE CONTAINER

Here is a script for a variation of this exercise, to shut down an incomplete session, or for somewhere to put other issues that came up to process later (Murray 2011; Shafer 2023):

1. "Please close your eyes or soften your gaze. We are coming to the end of the session and a lot of things came up today that we did not have enough time to address. So, I would like you to create a container of your creation to put in what feels unfinished or you want to put away for now to address later or at a future session."

2. "The size does not matter—it can be a famous building, a dresser with lots of drawers, the vault of a bank, a box of some kind. Remember, there is no right way or wrong way to do this."

3. Tell them there are just three rules about containers: "(1) The material they are made of is not see-through (we don't want anyone to be able to see what is in your container, only you). (2) We do not put people or animals in our containers, only our thoughts and feelings about them (we don't keep prisoners). (3) Please make sure there is a lock and key (a dead bolt with a combination lock or a keypad) so that no one can open the container except you."

4. Ask, "Do you have one?" (If they nod or say "yes," continue.)

5. "Now please put everything that feels unfinished from the session today in your container and when you are done, lock it shut and let me know by nodding your head or moving a finger." (Make sure you watch!)

6. "Now decide where you would like to keep your container; some like to keep it at my office, or a place in nature, or somewhere else the world."

7. Pause.

8. "Let me know when you are done by taking a long, slow exhale out through the mouth and opening your eyes."

9. First, ask how they feel, then ask them if they would like to describe the container and where they put it (to see if it "worked"). If they found this helpful they can close their eyes and see where they put the container; tell them they can use this exercise any time they get triggered or overwhelmed by something (thoughts), and they can use the container to put them there—and use the bilateral tapping to create the image and open the neural networks to "remember" they have a place to put stressful thoughts should they occur between sessions.

FOCUSING ON SENSATIONS

For most clients seeking out therapy, the most pressing question is: "How do I get rid of this?" or "What can you do to make it stop?" The fear of not being able to stop, change, or do something different can create anxiety or a sense of hopelessness. Yet, the insistence on the immediate elimination of this feeling or reducing the symptom is misguided. Freeing oneself of discomfort and anxiety is a valuable intention and an important part of healing, but, as we have seen, the symptom is only the tip of the iceberg, an indication of something else. It's equally important, and more valuable in the long run, to learn what the symptom means within the overall context of one's life. Only by turning toward the symptom and embracing it (which also involves going through and beyond the anxiety) are we able to release it and genuinely heal ourselves. And, yes, it is a lot of work and exhausting to pay attention and stay awake. Remember, you are not the symptom, and your intense emotions and thoughts are *real but not true now!*

Here is how to practice turning inward and toward focusing on sensation(s)/images.

Remember: You are not the symptom; your intense emotions and thoughts are *real but not true now!!!*

1. The next time you experience an intense emotion, sensation, or get triggered (and you will, because life is always challenging us to grow), instead of reaching for that drink, that joint, smoke, or engaging in some form of fight with a loved one or other trauma drama, *halt!* Stop and close your eyes.

2. Now focus on (just watch) the breath and notice the part of your body where you're feeling discomfort.

3. Name or label the symptom in any way you wish, whether that's *a headache, stomachache, worry, tightness, coughing, anxiety,* or [insert symptom here]. You name the visitor that is present.

4. See, sense, and focus on the message it is bringing you. Know that you are not the symptom (the anxiety, headache, etc.). You are you, and not that. That is a visitor, the brainbody trying to give you a message about what needs the power to wake up.

5. Remind yourself of this by saying aloud, or in your imagination: "Am I having FUN®?" If not, "What am I thinking about?" WAIT—"What do I need to Undo, and Now Act upon?" (For more information on this important aspect of the FUN® approach, see Chapter 2.)

6. See, sense, and feel how, by detaching from the symptom and the story, you create a space of freedom. Then slowly open your eyes.

7. Even if you can't immediately feel a separation from the intense emotion, stay with the symptom for up to a minute or two, just looking at it without telling a story, complaining, or running away from it. Know, for now, that *this is enough*—the ease of the intensity of sensation will calm down with practice. Try this whenever a symptom comes up, or as often as you can, without attaching to the outcome. Soon you will find that your ability to refrain from engaging or reacting to the symptom (or the genuine realization that "we are not the symptom") will begin to arise naturally, engaging your ability to self-regulate and control your nervous system. As you practice over time, you will distance yourself from cortically explaining the symptom, which, in turn, will give you a sense of release and relief.

Imagine what you can do with the brainbody therapies and exercises you now have to relax the nervous system. All you have to do is remain curious, go with that, relax, and have FUN®!

CHAPTER 9

Putting Your Healing Practices into *Action*—Future Training and Resources

The key to recovery, healing, and self-care is connection (we cannot do it by ourselves, but we must do it)—do not compare your journey or a client's "progress" to anyone else's. Everybody is sorting through something, so be kind to, considerate of, and compassionate with everyone. And remember, the brainbody is always curious, seeking pleasure, drama, and more information, while attempting to self-regulate.

As you continue to fall—and stay—awake, I suggest that you keep the following in mind: Change requires the Courage (and willingness) to do something different, Commitment to a daily practice, and having the Discipline to do it (Change = CCD). The essential tool for Falling Awake and living dis-ease free (going back to The FUN® Program and the First Session Exercise in Chapter 2, and the AIP model of EMDR in Chapter 3), is to *watch, listen, and keep paying attention*—with both the heart and the collective consciousness of your mind (the Committee you were introduced to in Chapter 2). To review, remember, the past is over, the future is being created as you live, and remain in the brainbody present *now*. And, yes, you can challenge beliefs, and I hope you revise or delete what is DEAD thinking (see Chapter 2) often, as the brain forest keeps growing and evolving, depending on which brainbody path you take.

Paying attention to your "symptoms" is a way of listening and attending to yourself—a self-care plan in action. To do this, it's necessary to step back a bit and stop analyzing, making up stories, overreacting, and judging. As we saw in Chapter 6, we are now noticing and changing our beliefs and behaviors—to move and do something different. This also involves not blaming, judging, comparing, or complaining about what is going on. Suspending this mental chatter (is the Committee running the show or am I thinking in a DEAD way?), even briefly, expands your awareness and cultivates a healthier outlook and relaxing way to live (even though a lot may be going on). The invaluable skill of becoming your own authority and taking a step back to notice what is going on in the brainbody forest will lead you on a healing journey that is far deeper than you might ever have thought possible. Remember, life is limitless but not for in perpetuity! Huh??? So, take heed and do the work! You have all the tools you need; please use them wisely or obtain professional help and training for guidance on how to implement them in your life and work with others.

Whatever path, practice, or therapy you choose for your self-care or for treating clients, how you keep your office, greet a client, land on a yoga mat, or prepare for a session, what you want from a session may impact the commitment to the brain forest journey, and how your clients connect and commit to their journey with you. Remember how we began in this book? Asking if your beliefs create your experiences or your experiences create your beliefs? The ability to literally "change your mind," that is, work with the neuroplasticity of the brain, requires inquiring about our motives, expanding our curiosity, and looking at how we respond to what is going on in our life (checking in on nervous system regulation—ventral–sympathetic–dorsal—as discussed in Chapter 1).

When asked about how we actually heal from trauma and other events that have impacted our lives, here is an observation of how Levine (2005) and Sovik (2005) describe the process: Trauma is about symptoms. It is what happens in our brainbody when we are exposed to extreme threat. Trauma responses are what happens when we become overwhelmed. Trauma and the responses to it, can, in fact, impact us in ways that don't show up for years. Something happens so fast and so quickly that the nervous system is unable to process it and restore our equilibrium. For example, a traumatized war veteran who jumps every time a car backfires is clearly responding to gunfire heard and exposed to in the past. Or a person who has suffered torture and confinement breaks out in a cold sweat or has a panic attack when riding on a crowded elevator, subway, or standing in the crowded pit at a Rolling Stones concert—it is easy to see the link. However, many, if not most, of us who have been overwhelmed by a series of less traumatic or dramatic events have responses that are not so obvious—but they can be big clues that open the treasure chest to reveal how the past may somehow be present.

When we keep reacting and engage in the trauma drama, we keep that amygdala fire burning and forget there is a whole world of neural networks available to access in the brain forest. These neurodivergent pathways are just waiting for us to explore them, or tend to them, to help us heal and be free—if we want to (we always protect our freedom to choose—remember the First Session Exercise in Chapter 2).

As I was writing this chapter, a client of mine, a young woman in her 20s, relapsed on crack and heroin—again. She had been in more than 20 inpatient treatment centers and was sober for over a year. This relapse began by her drinking alcohol while out at business parties over the holidays, and she found out her favorite aunt had just died. At the parties, she would sneak off to smoke crack in the bathroom "to hide her using." Her boss, who is 10 years clean and sober, told her she didn't need to detox or go to therapy (I believe this to be unsolicited advice, which is now also seen as an abuse of power at work)...she just needed to go back to meetings (AA/NA 12-step). The meetings do work for some people, but for an individual who has complex trauma, as she does, and who is a chronic relapser, there is a whole lot more going on than a 12-step program alone can offer. This is when the expertise of trained professionals—a team, a recovery tribe of healthy, sober "connections"—are so important in helping the person to stay on track. I am happy to say that this woman was able to get the help and support she needed, that miracles can happen every day, one day at a time.

According to Connie Zweig (2021, p.1), retired psychotherapist and author, "Age is our curriculum... Whatever age you are fellow traveler—Baby Boomer, Generation X, Gen Y (Millennial), or Gen Z—if you have opened this book (and made it this far into it), then you have heard the call."

By introducing you to the falling awake tools in this book, I do not mean to infer that you have to keep *doing more*. In fact, I am proposing just the opposite: Find the tools that work for you and the people you serve and use them (do less—stop searching for other solutions). During our lifetime, and as we continue to age, things will continue to happen to us. Like the neurodiversity of our brain forest, as we rewire and pull out the weeds, we discover emotional transformation is possible and can inspire others to do the same. When we fall awake, we transcend the borders of our imagination and become part of a greater emotional network that connects us with *all* living things (Forbes 2011).

> **If you're going through hell, keep going... (Winston Churchill)**

As implied by this quote, when your world feels like it is turning upside down again, here are some additional exercises to put in your falling awake toolbox.

IMAGERY FOR ANXIETY OR CONFUSION

Have a meeting with the Committee (the Monkey Mind). Bring all the parts of you to the table (Fraser 1991). These are all normal and are a part of you! They are a defense mechanism arsenal (also referred to as Protectors). Invite them to the table to discover which part holds the trauma, drama, protection, numbs out, or likes to gamble. Maybe there is the Codependent, the Victim, the Need for Drama part, the part that likes to have fun, or prance on the Red Carpet, the Acting Out/Rebellious Teenager, the Inner Child, the Rock Star, the Shamer, the Inner Critic, the Doubter, and so on. Spend some quality time with them. See what they have to say, and thank them for showing up and being with you all these years. Tell them how they can be helpful to you now.

For example, when the anxiety NFD part shows up, have a conversation or journal with the part to find out what is making them visit now. Remember, they are just doing their job to protect you; or it could be an old part from the past showing up because of something that is going on now. You can also go to an EMDR (The Pendulum, two-handed interweave) or Brainspotting therapist (find the brainspot to reveal the story) and explore what information needs to be accessed subcortically, or participate in a Yoga

Nidra session to invite this part with the intention of bringing all the anxious tension to awareness and letting it go (Hawkins 2012; Lasater 2007; Hanson Laster and Lasater 2009). You now have many ways to explore these parts of you!

Let's not forget your younger you part—as my colleague Insoo Kim Berg (1994), co-founder of Solution-Focused Brief Therapy, would say: "So!" To switch gears during the therapy session: How (you may be asking) do I start my healing journey? If you have a picture of your younger you, take it out and frame it and put it on your dresser. Every morning look at your younger you and say: "I love you—I have your back—Let me know if you need anything."

Keep on moving—and breathing

Our amazing self-healing brain and body is in a constant state of synaptogenesis (Badenoch 2008), which means new synaptic connections control the process of change and growth. Exercise and new experiences induce cells to split and create new ones in various areas of the brain, helping us learn new ways to self-regulate. Some "props" you can use to help the brainbody "land" in the therapy session and be curious are weighted blankets (for calming), holding a stuffed animal (to release stress or anxiety while talking), placing a warm or cooling wrap around the neck, or bouncing on a stability ball (to release trapped energy and correct posture). Other exercises to stimulate the brain anytime anywhere—and for distracting the looping mind—include listening to bilateral music, hula hooping/jumping jacks/elbow to knee, or just walking around the office (sometimes being outside can be helpful if appropriate too), to bring attention to the body and get out of the cortical thinking brain.

And, of course, if all else fails, you can always go back to focusing on the breath. Here are five qualities of the breath that you can explore for calming the emotions, quieting the mind, slowing the heart rate, and relaxing the body (just focusing on the breath does all these things): deep (propelled by firm and measured contractions of the diaphragm); smooth (flowing without jerks or agitation); even (with exhalations and inhalations approximately equal in length); without sound (flowing silently); and without pause (flowing with smooth and effortless transition between breaths).

- Close the eyes (if you like) and begin with a long, slow exhale (exhaling first immediately calms the brainbody).

- After the exhale, which engages the parasympathetic nervous system, take a short gentle inhale into the nostrils.

- As you inhale, feel the chest and belly expand (you can place a hand on the chest and belly to engage and focus on deep belly breathing).

- And then, without pausing the breath, begin to exhale and relax the belly, feel the chest relax, end with the air exiting through the nostrils—you can use a metronome on your phone or an actual one (the device produces an audible sound to slow down and count to, to distract the thinking mind—for example to a 4/6 count: 4 beats to the inhale, 6 beats for the exhale).

- Notice the breath is quiet, without sound.

- Do this for 5–10 rounds to obtain the benefits of calming the mind and relaxing the body.

- When ready, end with an exhale out through the mouth, relax the hands down, open the eyes (if they are closed), and take a moment to notice the effects, what you are feeling now.

When members of the inner chat room pop in for a visit, it might be time to strengthen preferred beliefs:

- "When thinking about all we/you have been working on, what can help you remember and stay connected to your preferred belief, how you see yourself now?" (Suggest a code word, maybe use a dry erase pen to write the word on the mirror: "Hello, gorgeous, precious being..." Or DNM (for drama no more), or just write "peace," "calm," or "be kind"...(or try the Scribble It Out exercise in Chapter 8).

- "What do you love or appreciate most about yourself?" (The Inner Critic may crash in on the session.) "When do you remember feeling the strongest love/appreciation for yourself?" Here you can tap that in (Chapter 3) or find the love/appreciation gaze brainspot (Chapter 4).

- "What do you want written on your tombstone?" (Various members of the Committee (see Chapter 2) may appear again.) "How are you living your life that way?" Whatever your client says gives you a very good indication of who they truly are (be aware of the mind-cortical chatter (also known as the Monkey Mind) that will try to override all this).

- "How have your trauma wounds shaped/disrupted your mission in life? What lessons have been learned?" Helping our clients find meaning in their wounds can help tremendously. I know that all my trauma/drama gave me gifts in life, and that is true for many.

- "What are your innate passions and desires? What is in your dream bucket?"

- For clients with a higher power, ask: "What would your Higher Power tell you is the truth about who you are, really?"

As you bring the session to a close, you can say something like:

We are almost out of time. You have done some very deep and profound work today, and I appreciate the effort you have made and for letting me hold the space for you, sharing it with all me. How are you feeling now? What have you learned today? What do you want to take away from our work today?

(If the answer seems helpful or healing you can tap it in; if not put it in the container to review next time—see Chapter 3).

Have FUN® and keep falling awake

I hope to have piqued your interest in falling awake, provided some new perspectives and practical tools, and sparked your interest in trying The FUN® Program and brain therapies presented in this book. I know from my own personal and professional experience that they work and that they can create lasting healing and change. Most importantly, trust *yourself—not the Wizard of Oz*, not your mother, husband, doctor, or other people you deem in power or "in the know," not even your closest friend. You alone know what works best for you—and you know when you are putting yourself on hold. When you become your own authority, the approval and agreement of others is no longer so important. How do you know when you are doing this? When the calm self is present and the mind is quiet.

I leave you with this invitation: Try some of the exercises in this book, engage in FUN® thoughts, kind words, and healthy behaviors, and practice using sankalpas or intentions (the motive watcher). Do the work, witness, sense, notice, and feel how your brainbody responds *now*. Over time, with repeated visits and practice, the results of your commitment, effort, and discipline will be revealed. All your work will reveal your truth and put a spotlight on what you may want to do differently or next. Maybe you will become a FUN® therapist like me, or just keep *falling awake*! Whatever you decide, choose to keep falling awake, stay curious, enjoy the journey, and just go with that...

Peace, So Hum, Jai Jai, Shalom, Ho!, Amen, Namaste...

May we all be happy, stay healthy, safe, sane, and don't forget to have FUN®...

CHAPTER 10

Debrief—Final Points
for Therapists

Now we begin with the end in mind and start again in the brain forest. Renowned for her research on the impact that guilt and shame can have on us, author Brené Brown (2018, p.240) put it this way: "When we have the courage to walk into our story and own it, we get to write the ending. And when we don't own our stories of failure, setbacks, and hurt—they own us."

Now that we are awake, I am offering some final suggestions for when your Committee starts challenging you and makes you wonder if you can try the new tools in this book. Here are some suggestions I was given along the way by my mentors and other therapists:

1.   Remember, you were a therapist before you used these tools and clients keep coming to see you. You already know what to do. Always trust your clinical judgment.

2.   Get to know and understand the client's core belief structure. (Ask: "As you think about or tell me this, what is the worst part?" Then you will have a memory or image.) Develop where to start from there.

3.   Know the developmental stages: "How old is this part, or when did this start?" Beliefs are verbal expressions of complex memories, feelings, and emotions about the past, things happening now, or anticipations about the future.

4.   Beliefs are evaluations of the self generally encoded along a developmental hierarchy during childhood. You can ask: "As you think about your childhood, what are your 10 best and 10 worst memories?"

5.   Trust the training in terms of the formats, setups, "protocols," and "scripts" provided to get you started. They are evidence-based. Embrace the uncertainty principle, stay in the "tail of the comet," WAIT, and see where it goes. You don't have to know why it is working, just know that it does.

6.   Implicit memories are nonverbal and developed in utero or infancy/childhood. The more dramatic, chronic, or intense, the earlier the encoding.

7. The timing of your intervention, comments, or feedback is done when you "feel" it is appropriate, necessary, or urgent. "Just do it." (We've all been there.) Offer comments at the end if the clients ask, or when there is a dead end ("Nothing is happening"), or if they want to stop. (Or try to "squeeze the lemon" by saying: "Notice you want to stop. There is information there for you, and go with that.")

8. When frozen in time, the stronger the threat (past, present, future), the more intense the fortress of the emotional encoding in the neural network (thoughts/feelings/sensations).

9. We all want to feel included and accepted. Check on connection to emotions. Existential: love for self and others. Relational: play/social activities. Secure: belonging/survival/safety.

10. And don't forget to help the clients consider: "Who am I? Why am I here? What do I want?"

11. If they say to you "I don't feel/notice/see anything" or "I can't remember," just say to them: "How does it feel that . . . . ?" Or, "That's great that you don't . . . . Just go with that/go from there."

And, of course, dear therapist, we are all fellow travelers, so please remember to take care of thyself—continue your falling awake process and have FUN®! Life is limitless, just imagine what you can do... Think about Lou Reed's "Walk on the Wild Side..."

Feelings Wheel

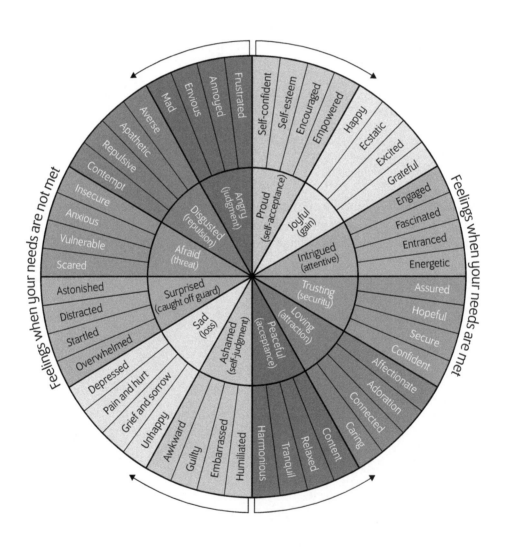

The FUN® Program

FUN® therapy: A comprehensive mindbody approach for behavioral health

Please see Chapter 2 for more in-depth information on The FUN® Program. Here you will find summary notes on its most important components.

Core concepts

- For a fun life, ask: What do I want? What do I need? Who am I?

- Freedom comes from the thoughts and choices you make. You have the power to make things happen—dare to be different.

- *Stay in the present*: The past is not so important. The Power is *Now*! When the mindbody is calm, attention is to every moment. Being awake and in control is a life of fun and ageless living.

- Take your MEDS: Mental imagery, Exercise, Diet, and Self-care.

- WAIT: Why Am I Talking? What Am Thinking? Why Am I Thinking?

- And perhaps WAIST: Why Am I Still Talking?

The FUN acronym

F = *Focus*—Pay attention/what you are thinking. What messenger is visiting?

U = *Undo*—Befriend the preferred beliefs/Committee/visitor

N = *Now*—What action needs to be taken?

The DEAD acronym

When the reactive mind (also known as the Monkey Mind or the Committee or the Inner Critic) is ignited, four types of thinking are involved in creating a DEAD head, which present as conflict, rage, fear, guilt, and separation, creating suffering and dis-ease:

D = *Denial*—Emotional hook: blame, anger, resentment (refusing to "take responsibility"). The "all or nothing" and "not me" syndrome. Avoiding some truth(s) about the present. Pointing the finger at everyone else.

E = *Expectations*—Emotional hook: worry, anxiety, panic, and fear. Making up stories, fortune telling (the "what if" syndrome). Also, creating standards that don't exist or labeling: "I'm a loser, bad mother/father, ugly," etc.

A = *Analysis*—Emotional hook: intellectualizing, attachment, ignorance. Always thinking (the "Mr. Know It All" obsession). Looking to authorities (like Google) instead of looking within, trusting your inner Oz that knows what to do.

D = *Doubt*—Emotional hook: sadness, regret, guilt, negative thinking. "It will never/won't work." The "would've, could've, should've" mental tapes, monkey mind, or cortical chatter tapes.

DEAD thoughts take you out of the present and engage the Committee. DEADly thinking puts the emotions in charge.

Members of the Committee (aka your protectors)

Accuser	Controller	Idol Worshipper
Addict	Coveter	Inner Critic
Arguer	Doubter	Inner Terrorist
Authority	Drama Queen	Inventory Taker
Awfulizer	Ego	Jealous One
Blamer	Expectations Expert (Standard Creator)	Judge
Caretaker		King Baby
CEO/Boss	Fearful One—The "What Iffer"	Know It All
Codependent	Fretter—Would Of/Could Of	Mind Reader
Competitor		Namer
Comparer	Helicopter Parent	Need for Drama
Concluder	Hypochondriac	Peacock (Pride/Vanity)

Perfectionist	Seeking Approval	Victim
Pleaser	Sensitive	Victimizer
Prisoner of War	Shamer	Whiner
Procrastinator	Skeptic	Workaholic
Protector	Social Arbitrator	Worrier
Rebellious Teenager	Storyteller	
Regretter	Wanting Attention	

Negative beliefs

Fake news + fake food + fake people are not FUN®! To live an authentically FUN® life starts with paying attention to what you are thinking about (WAIT). This means really looking at what you are allowing in, on, and around your mind and body (brain-body basics!).

Remember that all intense memories and reactive emotions are *real but not true now!* Undo the story. Somehow you may be making the past present. Practicing this makes *shifts happen!*

Here are five things to know about negative beliefs in addition to the fact that they are real but not true:

1. They multiply: what you practice, you strengthen.

2. They keep you from beliefing in yourself (Doubter).

3. They create obstacles for your success.

4. They do not make you feel happy.

5. You created them; it is a story you can edit and delete.

Try this for a calm, comfortable, secure present:

Inquire about the chatter—"How could he/she do this to me?" (blame); "I'm falling apart" (self-improve); "I'm not good enough" (people pleasing); or "I deserve better" (entitlement). "When I lose weight I will feel better" (self-improve); "I have to do it this way" (believing the Committee or someone else you are making an authority)... all conflict with doing what you want. Who is telling the story here? Did you pick up someone else's baggage?

Taking the first step is staying awake—being aware of the beliefs—and then undoing what has become the script since childhood: complaining, demanding, tantrums for control, blaming, pleasing for affect, obeying authority, feeling guilty, manipulation, lying, and self-improving. All these destructive ways of sticking to the story are exhausting you, can make you feel hopeless, and prevent you from being authentic and in charge of your life.

Yes, life can be stressful and challenging! Substance misuse, and other numbing-out behaviors such as food binging and restraining, alcohol misuse, smoking marijuana, gambling, watching porn, shopping, internet surfing, working all the time, shut up the Committee for a while, but when their effects wear off, the Inner Critic or other members emerge again and throw out the bait—guilt, shame, fear, drama, resentment—to see if you will "bite the hook" and continue to engage the habitual dialogue and numbing-out behaviors again, going back into that default mode network (DMN).

There is nothing wrong with pleasure. Everybody wants some attention, approval, the feeling of being useful, cared about, or loved—just feeling good! Physical pain, feeling ignored or rejected, feeling unwanted, or worthless can't always be avoided. All are grabbing our attention and visiting to give the message that something needs attending to. Emotional, mental, and spiritual pain are misunderstandings—situations that are part of life. Being awake and aware, these things don't become so painful, as the reactive mind starts calming down.

The first step for all human beings who wish to achieve their Limitless Potential is to understand that things do happen for a reason (I know you may not like to hear this). The work is to determine what this is and to own your part...this self-study is done without judgment, comparison, or the Inner Critic. Just observe as objectively as possible the purpose, motive, or intention of the action, belief, or situation: What is the benefit of the drink, the yelling, eating the whole cake, gambling away the rent, being a doormat, proving you were/are right, cursing and hanging up the phone, trying to control others? Just observe and notice if at some level the purpose is to control, gain pleasure, avoid pain, stop conflict—in spite of the consequences. This continuous self-study is the foundation of true unification and knowing you!

Remember you are important!!! Imagine what you can do!!!

> **The unexamined life is a waste of time. (Socrates)**

Life is a privilege—which can be taken away or end at any time, and without notice. We are in charge of our inner state and responsible for what we say and do. These cannot be taken away, but we often give them away.

Challenge yourself! Think like the person you want to be: younger, thinner, spontaneous, wild, free, happy. Enjoy the present, let go of control, find and retrieve, and "re-member" all the parts of you...all are welcome (Whitfield 1989). Remember yourself and become whole! This is your chance to ask questions, discover, and find answers. Start now by changing your routine, break habits. Life is a response calling you to take action, take charge, take responsibility, deprogram, and liberate—fall awake and have FUN®.

Laws of attraction: beliefs = experience

As you think, so you become. The addict/reactive mind makes the subject or situation the "God" or the "authority." Full attention is on being right, blaming, obtaining, using and/or recovering from the reactive state or the substance...which is about control. Codependency is granting authority to others: obey them, please them, walk on egg shells, or self-improve...all to avoid rejection or disapproval (the attachment/ addiction) from the perceived person (the problem). It is a subtle form of power over others to maintain verification that "I" exist. But you are, in fact, giving them the power.

When you dwell on what you don't want, or on what you don't have, or can't do, that is what is attracted. Pay attention to what you are thinking every moment. The mind, God, higher power, the universe, energy, whatever you believe, always responds to what is asked for all the time. It teaches us to be awake —and pay attention. Be the sheep dog. When we challenge beliefs and our stories, we force ourselves to recognize how emotions/thoughts/beliefs affect everything. We are then *awake*.

> *Imagine what you want. Imagination is more important than knowledge. Knowledge is limited while imagination embraces the world. (Albert Einstein)*

1. Ask for what you want, take charge—give it an image.

2. What answer do you get?—pay attention.

3. Be open to receive—beware of the Committee.

During the profound state of self-inquiry that takes place with YogaFUN® Nidra, the experience can be enhanced by developing a focus and anchor of stability and well-being that can be woven in at different points of the practice and throughout your day. Think about what you may want to work on during the next 4–6 months of your life. This brings you into the present by requiring you to take a moment to think about what you want right now in your life and alerting the Universe, God, or Goddess about how to wake up the neural pathways of the brain to assist with this. This is practicing in the state of awareness...welcoming in everything as it is without trying to change or "fix" anything. Accepting all as perfect, whole, and complete.

Ten suggestions for self-care

1. Relax more: "Remember that almost everything will work again if you just unplug it for a few minutes...including you!" (Anne Lamott,[1] American author and activist).

---

1   www.ted.com/talks/anne_lamott_12_truths_i_learned_from_life_and_writing

2. Each day, ask angels, archangels, winged beings, the goddess to open your heart. Remember—love is the most important ingredient.

3. Have FUN®! Use the program! What are you waiting for?

4. "Be open to the abundance of the world/universe/space around you and trust it is always there to give you what you want! The Universe has got your back." (Bernstein 2016)

5. Pay attention—be a thought watcher: WAIT.

6. Take time to just be: don't just do something...sit there!

7. Listen to music you love.

8. Go outside, see something beautiful. Move!

9. Read, keep the mind active and curious.

10. Eat fresh and clean! Cook!

Remember, as Anne Lamott said, expectations are resentments under construction. Change your frequency by embracing the emotions of love, relaxation, compassion, empathy, happiness, generosity, calm, ease, peace, connection. These will engage the FUN® way of living and being...

Say to yourself, "*yes*, I can! I am, I can, I will, I do, just *did*!" Remember to move, have FUN® and play music you love loud!

How to Create a Sankalpa, or Intention, with YogaFun® Yoga Nidra

How to choose a sankalpa or intention for the practice today

The following phrases are suggestions for what you may want to use for your focus during mindfulness practices like Yoga Nidra. You are also welcome to create your own! Essentially, it is a short statement of what you want your focus to be on, perhaps for the next 6–12 months, while you practice and in your daily life (when you wake up, throughout the day, and just before sleep).

A sankalpa or intention is a phrase you choose to say in the present tense, as though it is already happening. And as you establish this somatic, felt sense of intention, notice where and how you feel it in your body. There is no right or wrong way to create an intention for the practice. It is recommended you keep the same intention over time (remember, what you practice you strengthen).

I am at peace and am peaceful with others.
I bring light with me wherever I go. I see what is ahead. I am clear.
I am privileged and use this to empower others.
The actions I take in the world make a difference.
My recovery makes a difference in the world.
I communicate with kindness and compassion to myself and others.
I know when to speak and when to listen.
Unshakable confidence and trust breathes through me now.
I have everything I need to fulfill my life...it is already happening.
I am limitless.
I speak with confidence. My voice is worth being heard.
I communicate with others with kindness, consideration, and compassion.
I love my life. I am happy.
I love this body I have been given. I am privileged to have it.
I am comfortable with solitude. I feel at home with myself, my community, and the world.
Drama no more. I am grounded in peace. I pause before I respond.
I am loved. I am worthy of love.

I embrace my skills and talents and use them to achieve my purpose.

I know who I am and why I am here. I have teachers/spiritual advisors to guide me.

I know when to ask for help. It is okay to make my needs known.

I know whose advice to consider. I am open to constructive criticism.

I am present in every moment. I take one day at a time.

There is no rush to my transformation. It is okay to take my time.

I take time to breathe. It is okay to exhale and create space.

I can trust my inner wisdom. I learn from every moment. I have patience.

It is okay to change my mind. I can take time and consider my options.

I can let go of what does not serve me. I live in line with my values and ethics.

I am able to make changes in my life. I am adaptable. I believe in myself.

I have the inner resources I need to achieve my goals. I've got the power.

I am aware of my deepest desires. I am inspired. I dwell in possibility.

I find limitless potentials every day. I am clear on my goals and ambitions.

I take action every day to support my journey of recovery.

I am clear about my priorities.

I feel at home and relaxed in my body. I respect my body.

I treat myself with love, compassion, and respect. I am my best friend.

I meet and greet any and all changes or challenges with resiliency and openness.

I am strong, focused, and determined.

I am blessed with the freedom to create my life.

Words for living free, without drama

In creating your own phrase, here are some words you may want to consider:

> Teach Clean Leave Open Close Shut Sing Touch Practice Learn Focus Curious Breathe Relax Feel Watch Allow Notice Listen Surrender Watch Exhale Sense Calm Move Consider Align Soften Hold Support Release Yes No Fly Land Sit Stop Control Change Plant Clear Command Go Commit Enjoy Decide Choose Jump Remove Contemplate Understand Dump Shred Spin Dance Savor Imagine Love WAIT Peace FUN®

And words from the "A" list for further consideration

> Agni Awestruck Attentive Attuned Authority (be your own) Awake Amen A woman A man A being Amends Active Anonymous Alive Autonomy Alone Ability Animate Alive Ambitious Aloft Along Amazing Alluring Azure

The YogaFun® Yoga Nidra Script

Please see Chapter 5 for information on Yoga Nidra (see also Shafer and Desai 2023). Remember, it can be done lying on the back, on the side, or seated in a chair—whatever is most comfortable. If practiced in a chair, it is suggested to be backed up to a wall so the head can rest there if you doze off.

I created the YogaFun® Nidra Script, which has been adapted and used with permission from Kamini Desai to incorporate the brain.

Introduction

Welcome to "Falling Awake with Intention," the advanced relaxation session, also known as Yoga Nidra, which is the gold star for stress reduction, guided relaxation, and transformational awakening. Are there any newcomers to this practice? Any EMDR therapists, psychotherapists, or yoga teachers here? One of the most helpful mindfulness tools we can use is relaxation. In yoga, there are many such tools. This morning you are here to experience Yoga Nidra, which is different from Savasana (corpse pose), the relaxation practice that is done for a few minutes or as a guided meditation at the end of a yoga class.

Please make sure bracelets and watches, anything that can block your energy, is removed. Also please put all cell phones in the off position, as the buzzing in silent mode can distract you and others. Additionally, you may want to have a piece of paper and pen nearby so you can write down at the end of the class anything you wish to remember. This is for your use only. Go ahead and arrange for these now while I keep talking.

Yoga Nidra brings awareness into all that is possible in your life. It puts a spotlight on intense emotions, blocking beliefs and stories that may be holding you back in your life, and helps you transform these. This is a class on not only being present in the body and mind, but also allowing yourself to relax, and lie still on the floor fully awake, no movement required. Research on Yoga Nidra claims a 45-minute profound practice of relaxation, while remaining awake and alert throughout, is the equivalent of three hours of sleep! And while this is a session where you will not fall asleep, you might, however, have the experience of falling awake. Now negotiate with each other if you have their permission to nudge them slightly if they start snoring. You do not have the nudge them if you do not want to; we invite all noises here. For those of you on Zoom, we will not know if you are snoring unless you keep your sound on, so if you can hear me, please mute yourself now.

As I indicated earlier, while there are many approaches and theories to obtain the total experience of Yoga Nidra, please know this: there is no right way or wrong way to practice. Only your way. The focus of this morning's Yoga Nidra session will also integrate the sixth chakra (the third eye chakra), located at the center of the forehead, which is about trusting our intuition and expanding the imagination (and we all have one—no previous training required) (Judith 2015). The color of the sixth chakra is indigo, and the element is light, the light that is guiding us to see our way.

Opening stretches (optional)

Doing some Apana Kriyas (gentle stretching/exercises) can be helpful to balance the dosha (your temperament, vibration, energy) known as your nervous system. These gentle movements are also done to keep the joints and muscle tissues flexible, freshen the skin, and keep the internal organs functioning optimally, enabling you to lie or sit during the Yoga Nidra practice. Let's begin:

- Eye exercises

- Neck rolls/side stretch

- Shoulder rotation, 4–5 rounds (both directions)

- Toe/hand joints (make fists)

- Foot flexion

- Ankle rotation

- Leg raises/double-leg vibration.

Now make you way to the floor. Lying on your back, bring your knees to your chest, gently windshield wiper the knees to release the lower back, then extend the legs out; feel free to put a pillow or bolster behind the knees to provide support to the lower back.

Take a breath and as you exhale relax your arms and hands down, palms open towards the sky. Notice your left palm, right palm facing up. Place in the left hand what you want to release or let go of—make a gentle fist so you know it is there. In the right hand, place what you want to bring into your life, what you prefer to believe—make a gentle fist so you know it is there. Pendulate back and forth, going back and forth, slowly between the left hand and the right hand. Now experience what is in both hands at the same time. Notice what you are sensing now and where you feel this in your body—excitement, confusion, doubt? Just notice. Remember, there is no right or wrong way to do this, the brain figures it out all by itself. Just notice.

Take a breath, and as you exhale, relax the hands and the whole body fully.

If you are on your back, please bring your feet to the outer edges of your yoga mat. Allow your arms to rest away from the body, palms open to the sky. Now let all movement transform into stillness.

Now adjust your body so that you are completely comfortable lying on the floor. Separate your feet a little wider than your mat. Turn your toes outward and your heels inward. Place your arms and hands on the floor slightly away from your body, palms facing upwards, and your fingers lightly curled in a relaxed manner.

You may keep your head turned on to one side, or straight, nose toward the sky, whichever is most comfortable. Take care to see that your body does not touch any other object. You may cover yourself with a blanket if you are feeling cold and place an eye pillow or covering over your eyes if you wish. Make all the adjustments now so that you do not have to move for any other reason throughout the practice.

Yoga Nidra practice

Close your eyes gently. The entire practice of yogic relaxation will be done with the eyes closed. An eye covering can be helpful with this. As we begin, say to yourself, "I'm now going to practice Yoga Nidra. I will remain perfectly aware and alert throughout the practice." We will now begin the practice of Yoga Nidra.

Take a breath and let it go. Notice what is going on with you in your body and mind this morning. The Sanskrit name for this chakra is Ajna, which means both to perceive and to command. While we see images with our physical eyes, the third eye center (the place between the eyebrows) holds these images in memory, which can sometimes distort our perceptions about who we are. It is these perceptions that command our "reality." The purpose of Yoga Nidra, according to Yogi Amrit Desai, is to open this "Third Eye" that sees life at its core, permitting Divine grace to pass through and integrate in the human form. He says, "profound shifts can be initiated through this and it is only open and accessible to you during Yoga Nidra when you are deeply relaxed." It is here, at the third eye, that you are "free" from changing, controlling, or managing the experience. You actually get out of your way and "let thy will be done!"

Now bring your attention to the center between the eyebrows. Notice any sensations you may feel. Ajna means to perceive or command. It explores the life lessons that teach us about truth and wisdom and deepens our capacity to cultivate an internal dialogue, opening our mind to see beyond reason and understand beyond intelligence. The color of this energy center is indigo—deep blue; the element is light. Through the Ajna chakra, we learn about intuition, imagination, insight, thought, vision (images), and self-evaluation.

Think about your intention this morning as you focus on the sixth chakra. Some of the questions you may want to consider as we go into Yoga Nidra are: are you willing to access the powerful knowing that is available to you? Such as: do you trust your intuition? Are you seeing a pattern? Can you see the big picture? Do you trust your inner voice? Can you trust your insight? Ask for Yoga Nidra to help you explore these.

Perhaps you already have a sankalpa or intention that you use for your own practice; if you do, please feel free to use that. If you do not have one for this practice or would like one, do go along with the power of the third eye or the sixth chakra. Perhaps it could be: "I allow intuition of my mind and body to create a profound healing shift now." Or: "I trust my guides to show me the way." Or: "I am limitless, I am at peace with myself and the world as it is, I am free." Choose what feels correct for you and repeat these words to yourself if you like, three times.

Feel every cell of your body receive the vibration or words of your intention. Imagine, see, sense, and notice three circles of light surrounding your body. These circles of light create a cocoon of comfort and protection around your whole body. Now allow yourself to be completely grounded in your body. Detach yourself mentally from any distracting thoughts that may arise in your mind. Even if you momentarily get carried away with a thought or a distracting noise, never mind, just come back to the instructions with relaxed awareness.

Right now, try to notice and bring your attention to hear sounds coming from a distance. There are several sounds that you may can hear. Don't think about them, just listen to them passively. Now gently allow yourself to concentrate on the sounds coming from inside this room alone. Let the sounds from outside fade out of your consciousness. You are practicing yogic relaxation. Be aware of each and every sensation that arises in your body.

Take a long, slow and deep breath. Breathe out completely. And as you breathe out imagine all your tensions, worries, flowing out of your body. Breathe in, slowly and completely, and as you breathe in, imagine all the vital energy from outside fill you on the inside. Breathe out, slowly and completely. As you breathe out, your tensions, worries are getting washed out of your system.

Once again, breathe in, energy flowing in; breathe out, tension flowing out. With each breath that is passing out, your body is relaxing further. As you settle in notice and feel the support of the Earth beneath you. Your whole body being held by the Earth on the floor.

Lie back, relax your body, deepen your breath. Parts of the body impacted by the third eye chakra are the brain, the neurological system, pituitary gland, pineal glands, the eyes, face, ears, and sinuses. Close your eyes and allow yourself to land here and quiet your mind.

Be still.

The questions we might explore around this chakra are about wisdom, discernment, knowledge, imagination, and intuition.

Ask yourself: How wise do you feel about your life right now?

Ask: Do you listen to your knowing and follow its guidance? Does your knowledge or wisdom get in the way of your experience at times? How do you utilize your imagination?

Ask: What about your intuition? Are there attitudes, ideas, or beliefs that have stopped you from trusting this?

Take a breath and exhale deeply.

Now let go of thinking. There is no where you have to go, nothing to do. Just be here, right now, in this moment.

Relax, trust, and let go...

Breathe in fully and exhale with a deep sigh. Again, breathe in fully and let go even more. Give yourself permission to breathe in the word "let" and exhale the word "go."

Now bring your intention for this morning's practice into your awareness again. If you are unclear about your intention, just see what happens as you lie here in your field of awareness. Repeat this intention silently to yourself three times. Or repeat these words: "I allow the intuition of my mind and body to create a profound healing shift now." Feel every cell of your body receive these words: "I allow the intuition of my mind and body to create a profound healing shift now."

Four breaths

We will now move our attention to the body to release trapped energy, tension, and charged emotions, and move more deeply into total relaxation. Remember, if you have any pressure in the head for any reason or are pregnant, it is important that you breathe normally as we go through the following tense and release exercises.

Upper body

As you inhale make fists and deliberately induce stiffness and tension throughout your shoulders, arms, and fists. Tighten, tighten, even more. Now let go completely and relax with a sigh.

On your next exhalation, relax even more.

Now let go completely. Reeeeelaaaaaxxxxx...

Observe, sense, and feel the flood of energy in your arms, left and right.

Lower body

This time, as you inhale, deliberately induce a feeling of stiffness and tension in the hips, legs, and feet. As you tighten, tighten, hold, hold...

And let go. Relaxxxxxxx...and let go completely.

Observe the flow of energy in your lower body now: the hips, both legs, both feet. Observe and sense the flow of energy in your legs.

Take 3 breaths.

Whole body

This time tighten and tense the entire body as you inhale: arms, hands, shoulders, feet, legs, face, buttocks, tighten, tighten, hold, hold...

Now exhale and let go completely. Reeeeelaaaaaxxxxx...

On your next exhalation, let go even more.

Observe and feel the flood of energy extending to all the muscles, nerves, and cells of your entire body. Pause.

Let your whole body melt into the flood of energy you feel in your body. Pause.

Let your whole body go limp, like a rag doll. Relax even more. Pause.

Release any holding, anywhere. Pause.

Take 4 breaths.

Instruct

Maintaining this inner stillness, see if you need to cover yourself, cover your eyes, or use any other props to make you feel even more comfortable. We now begin the practice of Yoga Nidra. Remain as motionless as possible. If you need to move or make an adjustment for any reason, please do so mindfully and return to stillness as soon as you are able. Resolve to remain awake, staying in touch with the sound of my voice. Allow your entire body to respond to my words directly, without thinking or analyzing. Allow any disturbances or sounds outside or inside this room to draw you inside more deeply. During Yoga Nidra, you enter the subconscious pranic field.

Let your mind merge and melt into the energy body and go beyond the boundaries of body and mind.

Now shift from thinking and doing to feeling and being. Pause.

Do absolutely nothing from now on. Simply reeeelaaaax...

Drop into the deepest state of tranquility, stillness, and peace at the third eye center...

Take 4 breaths.

Induct: complete yogic breath

Now follow my guidance as we begin the relaxation breath.

Breathing in deeply, fill your lungs from the bottom to the top, as if you are filling a water bottle.

As you breathe out, empty the lungs from top to bottom.

Let your breath be slow and steady.

Observe the movement of your abdomen and chest.

Stay connected to the wonderful feeling with the release of tension and the deep feeling of relaxation.

Let this feeling extend to every part of your body.

Now redirect your full attention to your breath.

Slowly deepen your inhalations and exhalations.

Let the flow of your breath be steady and uniform as much as possible.

Bring your undivided attention to your breath.

Slowly deepen your inhalations and exhalations.

Let the flow of your breath be steady and uniform as much as possible.

Bring your undivided attention to the movement of your abdomen and chest as you breathe in and out. Pause.

With each breath out, release any tension held in your body and anticipations in the mind. Let it all go. Just let go.

With each breath that you inhale, fill every nerve and cell with pulsating, healing energy.

Relax and pause for a few breaths.

Breathing out, let go of holding anywhere in your body. Let go even more.

Empty the body and mind and enter deeper levels of stillness and silence.

Pause.

Now breathe normally and be still.

Let all tension simply melt, drain away, and dissolve in the expanding energy field. Bring your attention to your eyebrow center... Recognize your deep connections to the original source of life force. The life energy that sustains your life and is an extension of your soul.

Take 4 breaths.

Integrate: dropping into being

Drop into that silent space where all doing stops. Pause.

Let go. Let go even more. Pause.

Enter an effortless state of being.

Notice what you are sensing in your body now.

Take 4-to-6 breaths.

We now begin the imaginary journey around the body.

Let us become deeply aware of each and every part of the body. This imaginary journey around the body is to help us focus and experience every sensation that arises in every part. As we focus on that part and relax it mentally, we then move ahead.

Follow my guidance as we move through different parts of the body. Let your attention rest on each body part as I name it, without comment or judgment:

- All 10 toes

- Both ankles

- Both knees

- Pelvis

- Abdomen

- Chest

- Arms

- Hands

- Throat

- Face

- Back of the head

- Shoulder blades

- Spine

- Buttocks

- Calves

- Heels

- Soles of the feet.

Sense the whole body from the top of the head to the tips of the toes. Whole body, whole body in awareness. Feel the whole body contained in vast, spacious awareness. Pause.

Now as I name each organ, feel energy moving with attention, nourishing and vitalizing each organ. Even if you don't know where the organs are, your brain and body does. Bring your attention to the:

- Heart

- Lungs

- Esophagus.

Left side of the torso, bring your attention to:

- The stomach

- Pancreas

- Spleen.

Right side of the torso, bring your attention to:

- The liver

- Gall bladder.

Now the abdomen, bring your attention to:

- The adrenal glands

- Kidneys

- Intestines

- Reproductive organs

- Bladder.

Now as we make our way up to the brain, sense and feel energy moving with attention, nourishing and vitalizing this epicenter of our neurology. Even if you don't know where these nervous systems are and what they do, your brain and body does.

Pause.

Place you focus and attention on the spinal cord, the super sensory highway beginning at the bottom of the lower back between the hips. Sense the spinal cord as a command center, sending sensory information from the whole body up the spinal cord to the brainstem at the base of the skull. Feel the energy from the spinal cord accessing all the chakras from the lower back up the spinal cord to the crown of the head and beyond, coordinating and balancing all the muscles, bones, and neuropathways, including the parasympathetic and sympathetic nervous system located at the brainstem at the base of the skull.

Pause.

Now bring your attention to your head and neck softening, easing.

Bring your attention to the back of the head.

Accessing the base of the skull, sense the limbic regulating region of the brain. Within this area, find the hippocampus, where our emotions and memories are stored and retrieved. Sense the thalamus, the relay station where some of the senses are involved in interpretating and learning information received. Refresh these regulation centers of the brain that provide information to the amygdala (known as the alarm center), programmed to react about our past or when we are in danger or be at rest in the present in trust, safety, and peace.

Pause.

Now bring your attention to the face.

With your next exhalation, allow all expression to drop from the face.

Releasing the tiny muscles around the eyes, within the eyes, the retina, allowing the eyeballs to rest back into their sockets.

Releasing the tiny muscles around the mouth.

The jaw.

Tongue resting in the mouth.

Sensing the cheeks.

Both ears.

Space between the ears.

Pause.

Now focus your attention to the point between the eyebrows and about three inches into the center of the brain.

Pause.

Sense the pituitary, the master gland, returning hormones to balance and harmony.

Pause.

The hypothalamus, allowing the entire nervous system to rest and reset.

Pause.

The pineal gland, rejuvenating body and mind, syncing your internal rhythm with the rhythms of nature.

Pause.

Prefrontal cortex, just behind the forehead, strengthening emotional intelligence, empathy, and compassion.

Pause.

Left hemisphere of the brain, involved with curiosity, logic, and reason restored to clarity and objectivity.

Right hemisphere of the brain, associated with creativity, imagination, and inspiration naturally blooming within the brain.

Now sense all the neurons and neuropathways in the brain at the same time. Neurotransmitters optimally flowing, communicating, connecting every part of the brain with every other part of the brain.

Scalp, resting on the skull, protecting the brain.

Pause.

Simply be available to the entire range of sensations in the head, face, and brain.

Pause.

Now bring your whole body into awareness. Feel the whole body contained in vast, spacious awareness.

Pause.

Notice the hollow notch at the base of the throat.

Notice sensation in the right rib cage, torso, hip, thigh, kneecap, and the hollow space behind the knee, shin, ankle, all the way down to the hollow space at the sole of the foot and all the little bones in the toes. Sensation flowing through the whole right side of the body. Whole right side of the body, radiant, spacious, hollow, and empty. Feel the whole right side of the body lying on the floor. The energy field radiant, shimmering around the right side of the body lying on the floor.

The hollow notch at the base of the neck.

Now breathe your way over to the left side of the body. Awareness of sensation. Bring your awareness to sensation in the left shoulder, all the way down the arm to the hollow spaciousness in the palm of the hand and all the little bones in the fingers, and the tips of the fingers.

Notice the hollow notch at the base of the throat.

Notice sensation in the left rib cage, torso, hip, thigh, kneecap, and the hollow space behind the knee, shin, ankle, all the way down to the hollow space at the sole of the foot and all the little bones in the toes. Sensation flowing through the whole left side of the body. Whole left side of the body, radiant, spacious, hollow, and empty. Feel the whole left side of the body lying on the floor. The energy field radiant, shimmering around the left side of the body lying on the floor.

The hollow notch at the base of the neck.

Now breathe into both sides of the body simultaneously. Become aware of both sides of the body. Awareness now of the whole body lying on the floor. Whole body resting, breathing, lying on the floor.

Now we drop down and experience the sense of feeling heavy and light.

Heavy

As I name the body part, bring your total attention there, accompanied by a feeling of heaviness, sinking, like a stone in water:

- Both feet, heavy and sinking, like lead weights.

- Calves and knees, heavy, and sinking deeper.

- Thighs and hips, very heavy. Like lead.

- Abdomen, chest and back. Gravity pulling you down, deeper.

- Shoulders, arms and palms. Very, very heavy.

- Feel your entire head, heavy like a stone.

Give your body completely and totally to the omnipresent field of gravity. Pause.

Now experience your whole body heavy like a rock.

Feel your whole body sinking deeper and deeper. Totally letting go, into the pull of gravity. Sinking, sinking, heavy like a stone. Sinking deeper into stillness and silent awareness.

Pause. Take 3 breaths.

Light

Now shift your attention, and as I name each part of the body, let all the heaviness drain away. Let your body be buoyant and light, like a fluffy cloud:

- Both feet, limp and light.

- Calves and knees, empty and free. Feel it.

- Thighs and hips, hollow and empty.

- Abdomen, chest, and back, light and empty.

- Shoulders, arms, and palms, floating.

- Head, hollow and empty.

- Feel your whole body empty, light and hollow.

Sense the emptiness of your body and the silence of your mind.

Pause. Take 3 breaths.

Energy body (optional)

Enter the power and protection of your energy body.

Embrace its feathery lightness.

Feel completely safe and secure.

Feel yourself getting lighter and lighter until you begin to float in the air.

Give yourself permission and freedom to float out of your physical body.

Release your energy body from your physical body.

Feel released and freed from identification with your body and mind.

Pause.

Observe your body completely at peace and resting in stillness.

Recognize you are spirit or energy separate from the physical body.

Enjoy this sensation of being limitless and free. The innate healing wisdom of the body, liberated, free, and functioning optimally on its own. Pause.

Now settle back into the physical body as you remain deeply established in your connection with spirit, faith, energy, and trust.

Take 4 breaths.

Integrate (choose several)

Resting in awareness at the center of the forehead, bring your awareness to the center between your eyebrows and drop into the deepest level of relaxation. Here there is nothing to do or achieve; you have entered the domain of limitless grace where anything and everything is possible.

Notice and allow any feelings and emotions present right now as you focus on this energetic layer of the body. Back of the body heavy, sinking into the earth like stone in sand. Legs heavy and sinking. Spine, back of the head, arms, heavy and sinking.

Now, very gently, allow any painful memory to emerge in your mind. Any event that was truly painful for you. Imagine that event and allow yourself to reexperience that pain.

Pause.

You are, in fact, reliving that event. Once again, take a long slow and deep breath. And as you breathe out, allow your skull, forehead, and face to relax. Let the shoulders relax. Allow your back, abdomen, and pelvis to relax. And say to yourself: "I am willing to let go. I release fear. I release anger. I release guilt. I release sadness. I release. And now I am at peace."

Pause.

Now allow the mind to recall another memory. This time something that made you happy. Bring forward any pleasurable event. Allow this to emerge in your consciousness.

Pause.

Imagine and see it clearly. Sense and feel the joy all over again. Pause.

And now release this too. Gently. Now say to yourself: "I am the creator of my life. I am an open channel of creative energy. Thoughts no longer have any power over me. I have power over my thoughts." Pause.

"I have the power to choose to feel and think the way I want." Pause.

In this highly powerful state of mind, imagine and visualize something powerful and wonderful that you want to have happen in your life. Pause.

Imagine and see, sense, and feel this clearly. Build on this image and see it in all its detail. Touch it. Feel it. Hold the image in your awareness and your heart. Feel joyous all through you as you picture and see you in this image. Pause.

You are feeling an abundance of immense joy. Now say to yourself: "This, or something better, manifests for me now, in totally satisfying and harmonious ways for the highest good of all concerned." Repeat: "This, or something better, manifests for me now, in totally satisfying and harmonious ways for the highest good of all concerned." Because of the highly potent state of consciousness that you are in right now, what you are imagining and dreaming of right now in this practice will come true in your life. Pause.

With a lot of contentment in your heart, let this image dwindle slowly. You have now accessed the deepest part of you. This is the state of having that sense of connection or purpose with the world. It is conceived of the finest veil in which you are feeling a connection to the Divine, a sense of wholeness, of feeling complete. Pause.

Remain empty and free from all doing.

Feel yourself as time transcendent presence, now.

Take 8–10 breaths in silence.

Intention

Here your intention and what you want to happen in your life are being actualized and fulfilled with effortless ease. Bring this to your attention and say your intention to yourself again now. You may also use, "I allow my body to create a profound healing shift now." Pause.

Allow this intention to go to the deepest levels of consciousness without hesitation. There is no need to do anything about it.

Bring your attention back to the third eye center (the sixth chakra) between the eyebrows and feel all the energies of your body...all the meridians activated, purified, and balanced.

Take 4 breaths.

Affirmations (choose three)

Allow your entire self to respond spontaneously and without effort to what I say.

"I return to the innate wisdom of my body to heal itself. I remain in restful awareness. I relax so completely and let go so fully that the inner healing blueprint of my body functions freely and optimally. Now that I have entered the deepest levels of letting go, I have entered a complete state of synergy and balance."

Take 4 breaths.

You are the vessel, the container of light and love. Carry it everywhere you go and share with everyone you meet.

If you have an area you feel needs healing, physical, mental, or emotional, allow this light and love of the sixth chakra knowing to flow into that area now.

Take 4 breaths.

Externalize

Now begin to become aware of the rising and falling of the breath. Pause.

Slowly feel yourself beginning to rise to the surface of awareness. Pause.

Disband, release, and let go the three circles of light surrounding your body. Let them go. Notice what you are sensing in your body now Sense the body resting on the floor completing relaxed all this time. Pause.

Notice the quality of the air as it touches the skin. Pause.

Now be aware of your nostrils. Air going into the right, exhale to the left.

Become aware of your head and face. Your legs. The muscles of your chest and abdomen. The muscles of your back. Your right hand, from the shoulder to the finger tips. Your left hand. Both legs. The right leg, from the thigh down to the toes. Your left leg.

Try and make gentle movements of your fingers and your toes. It may feel very difficult initially. But persist, gently, at it. Move your hands and legs a little more. Stretch your hands and legs completely.

Stretch your whole body thoroughly.

Bend your knees and bring them toward the chest and gently rock both and forth gently. Take your time, do not hurry.

Then just turn gently onto your right side and pause here for a moment with the eyes closed.

Feel the safety, comfort, and protection and insight of the third eye center (the third chakra).

Bring your intention into your awareness now again, changing nothing, silence.

"I allow my mind and body to create a profound healing shift now," or whatever you wish to say to yourself.

Every time you find yourself in reaction, you are empowered to replace it with your intention.

With your eyes remaining closed, gently use the top hand and arm to gently push you up into a seated position. Whatever seat is comfortable for you.

Sit up tall, make gentle fists with your hands, and gently tap your head to wake up the brain. Rub your palms against each other. Cover your eyes with your palms. Open your eyes inside your palms. Become aware of the light surrounding you. And gently place your hands together at the third eye center.

As the Ajna chakra develops, we become more intuitive, perceptive, imaginative. Allow this space to open. Find the courage now to open more fully into the wondrous mystery of being the fabulous being you are.

Continue to stay deep in this deep inner experience. Allow your hands to drop down, keeping the eyes closed if you would like.

Regardless of what you consciously recognize about what has or has not changed, know that something deep within has shifted to connect you with your intention.

Become aware of your body, and bring a deep sense of peace and contentment with you as you bring attention back to the body.

Notice how relaxed the body is now, how soft the breath is, how silent the mind is, how calm the heart beat is. Be still and be grateful. Know that you can easily enter here again and again.

Now when you are ready, open your eyes.

Feel the stability of your seat and lengthen your spine.

Place your hands at your heart center.

We meet here tonight as fellow soul travelers, we meet as living and loving beings, treating each other with kindness and nice cream.

Albert Einstein said in 1929: "Imagination is more important than knowledge. For knowledge is limited, whereas imagination embraces the entire world, stimulating progress, and giving birth to evolution."

This brings us to the end of our practice of Yoga Nidra. Thank you for joining me and falling awake with intention. May we all be happy, healthy, safe, sane, and have FUN®. Namaste.

61 Points Exercise

This exercise is adapted from Sovik (2005) and Desai (2017). To begin, lie on your back on a firm, flat surface. Use an eye pillow to cover your eyes if you like. Separate your legs a little more than hip width apart. Draw your shoulder blades underneath you with your arms about 8-to-10 inches out next to your side, palms up. If necessary, place a bolster or a blanket underneath your knees to relieve any back strain. Close your eyes and let your body rest and feel supported by the Earth beneath you. You can hear the sounds around you as they come and go with each passing moment. You can also sense the space around you. Gradually, let go of other times and places and rest in this moment in time.

Now bring your awareness to your body. Feel the back of your body feeling the surface and allow the weight of your body to settle down and land into this moment. Sense the front of your body. Picture yourself lying in a meadow or another place in nature on a warm Spring day. Your body is bathed in the sunlight and relaxes. Sense the outside of your body, the touch of the air against your skin, and the clothing surrounding you. Now gently go inside, and sense and feel your body from your head to your toes. Now bring your attention to your breath and feel the movement of your breathing. The breath flows out, and then flows in, again and again. As it flows out, it empties. You release and let go all feelings of fatigue, strain, and emotional tension. As the breath flows in, you are drawing in fresh energy and a sense of well-being and peace. Bring your awareness to the belly region. Softening there let the abdomen rise as you inhale and fall as you exhale. Breathing out, the abdomen falls and the lungs empty. And you release tension. Breathing in, the abdomen rises and the lungs fill, and you are nourishing the body with fresh energy.

Now continue to feel the movement of the abdomen. And gently breathe without pause between the breaths. Let each breath flow into the next in a smooth, unbroken stream. Finally, relax your effort to breathe. Let the breath flow easily and smoothly. You are the inner witness, feeling the inner flow of your breathing, and yet remain relaxed.

Now gently relax from the crown of your head to the bottom of your feet. Then travel from your toes through your legs to the base of your spine and relax from the base of your spine back to the crown of the head. And breathe as if your entire body breathes. Cleansing and nourishing with each breath, all your body to relax and rest... feel at peace right now in this moment.

Now begin moving through the 61 points. The first point is the eyebrow center and rest there. Sense a blue starlight point of energy. See, sense, and feel this blue star resting at this point as you breathe out and breathe in. Now shift your awareness to the throat center. Again, sense this starlight point of energy, blue star resting as you feel the flow of your breathing and the body relaxing. Now shift your awareness to the right shoulder joint. Right elbow. Right wrist. Blue starlight point of energy at the tip of the right thumb. Index finger. Middle finger. Ring finger. Small finger. The right wrist. Elbow. Shoulder. Throat center. The left shoulder joint. Left elbow. Left wrist. Tip of the left thumb. Index finger. Middle finger. Ring finger. Small finger. The left wrist. Elbow. Shoulder. Throat center. Travel down to the heart center. Right breast. Heart center. Left breast. Heart center. Naval center. Pelvic center. The right hip. Right knee. Ankle. Tip of the large right toe, second toe, middle toe, fourth toe, small toe. The right ankle. Knee. Hip. Pelvic center. The left hip. Left knee. Ankle. Tip of the large left toe, second toe, middle toe, fourth toe, small toe. The left ankle. Knee. Hip. Pelvic center. Naval center. Heart center. Throat center. Eyebrow center.

Rest and breathe, sensing all these points. Your body is like a space, a cosmic space filled with light and energy. In this field of stars. Your breath is like the wind filling and emptying all the spaces within your body as your awareness fills this vast space. Body resting, breathing, letting the breath pass in and out without effort. You are filled with the sensations of these points filled with blue starlight energy as you feel and sense each breath. And as you continue to feel the flow of your breathing, relax your mind. Your mind is like an inner space in the space of your mind. This space of your awareness is filled with the quiet sensations of the breath. You are the inner witness, relaxing your body, breathing, and mind.

When you are ready, gently breathe a little deeper, gradually sensing the space around you. Feel the quietness in that space. Same as the space within you. Then slowly bring your hands to your face and slowly massage your face. Then cup your hands over your eyes and open your eyes into the palms of your hands. Draw your awareness into the space around you. Gradually roll to your side and, after resting there for a moment, come back to a sitting posture. Gently tap the head.

Place your hands together at the heart center. Om, peace, peace, peace.

Becoming your own loving parent

This exercise is adapted from Twelve Steps from Adult Children of Alcoholics® & Dysfunctional Families. Mother's Day, Father's Day, holidays, and other days reminds us how parents and caregivers spend an extraordinary amount of time taking care of both the physical and emotional needs of others, especially children—or not, depending on what we experienced during different stages of our childhood and adolescence. The whole concept of loving ourselves (depending on what became our normal as children) is often ignored and our own personal needs and feelings are put on hold. It's not typically a conscious act, but this type of self-neglect can have a negative effect on our health. Imagine how much better we would feel if we turned some of that same love and attention to ourselves, becoming our own loving parent. It's the ultimate in self-care!

The most important first step in becoming a loving a parent is awareness, and one of the best ways to achieve awareness is through self-care practices like Yoga Nidra. While yoga is commonly thought to involve a series of poses on a mat, the benefits of achieving focus and a calm state can also be attained by simply lying down and relaxing (remember, no headstands and pretzel twists required).

On Mother's Day, Father's Day, and other holidays that involve parents and parenting, beyond all the lovely lunches, dinners, family gatherings, and time at the spa, take a few moments to be a good parent to yourself. Practice self-love, do a little yoga, and remind yourself how amazing you truly are! And remember EMDR, Brainspotting, and The FUN® Program can also help you wake up, recognize, and release those intense emotions and complex memories that have been lying dormant...time to wake up, let go, and be free... Namaste.

Resources to Use When Triggered or You Start to Go into Overwhelm

The Container

Sometimes when we have so much on our mind, or if it is the end of a therapy session and we need to shut things down "for now," we need a place to put these issues and return to working on them another time—this is where the container you create in your imagination can be helpful. Your container can be as big and elaborate as you want, or it can be the size of a jewelry box—here size does not matter!

There are, however, four suggestions about the container you choose: (1) Whatever material your container is made of, make sure it is not see-through—so only you know what is in your container. (2) You have a way to lock it shut with the lock of your choice, such as a padlock, combination lock, or a code that only you know, so when you are finished putting all you want in there you can lock it shut. (3) It is suggested we do not put people or animals in the container (we do not take prisoners or hold beings hostage), just our thoughts and feelings about them. (4) When you are finished putting all aside for now and have locked it up, now put it somewhere where you know it will be until you are ready to work on them again. This can be left at the therapist's office, out in a place of nature (bottom of the ocean, in a famous building, buried in the woods, etc.), or someplace in your home. You decide. And when you are ready to come back to the present moment, just breathe out through your mouth slowly and open your eyes.

Notice how you are feeling now.

The Four Elements Exercise

This exercise is adapted from Elan Shapiro (2012). Please find a comfortable seat, such as on a chair (feet on the floor) or on the floor—whatever seat is most comfortable for you—and just land right now, here, in this moment. Take a reading of your stress level at this moment on a scale of 0–10, where 0 is no disturbance and 10 is the highest you can imagine.

Now acknowledge yourself for taking the time to do this practice of self-care, for taking time out for you. We have many choices for how to spend our time, so give yourself credit for making this time for you. We are about to do what is called the Four Elements Exercise. The four elements are the Earth, Air, Water, and Fire. This will take about two minutes (the anxious/fidgety types will appreciate you telling them this so they do not think they will be here for 20 minutes). Please close your eyes, if you are comfortable, or just soften your gaze toward the floor. There is no right way or wrong way to do this exercise, only your way.

We will begin with the first element: Earth. Take a moment to notice how you are supported by the Earth, starting with your feet, if you are seated on a chair, or your tailbone if you are on the floor. However you are seated, just notice how your whole body is supported and held by the chair, or the floor, which is resting on the Earth beneath you. You can wiggle your toes if you like and gently rock back and forth from side-to-side, knowing the Earth is always there to support you.

Now bring your attention to your breath and the second element, which is Air. Notice the Air gently going in the nose and out through the nose or mouth. Focus on longer exhales out, shorter exhales in through the nose to engage the relaxation response. As you breathe out imagine any and all stress you may be experiencing leaving your body, making room for calm, relaxing Air as you inhale (pause). In fact, if you like, you can inhale the word "let," and exhale the word "go." Notice how more you feel relaxed when you give yourself permission to let...go...

Now bring your attention to your mouth. Notice the saliva inside your mouth, also known as Water, which is the third element. Sometimes when we are feeling stressed or anxious the mouth dries out. To increase the Water in your mouth, gently move the tongue around. Massage the upper gums, lower gums, move the tongue all around to create more Water. This is also to let the brain know that you are not in a fight, flight, freeze, or faint response. Everything in this moment is calm, secure, and at ease.

Now for the fourth element, which is Fire. Allow the Fire to light up your imagination (everybody has one), to bring up an image of a place you have been before or have seen in a magazine or a movie, or a memory that made you feel happy. Know that you can go back here anytime you close your eyes to feel peaceful, calm, and relaxed (pause). And if no place comes to mind, just see the word "peace" or the word "calm."

Now take a reading of your stress level now on a scale of 0–10 (0 = no stress, 10 = a great deal of stress). What do you notice now? If you are feeling better, you can tap this in, if you wish, to enhance the sensations you are feeling now.

The Four Elements Exercise integrating the Inner Resource System (IRS)

Take a moment to land where you are and acknowledge and congratulate yourself for taking the time to take care of you. We will begin with a grounding exercise called the Four Elements Exercise and help you find your Inner Resource System, your inner "IRS" that will be created by you as your recovery tribe. The four elements are Earth, Air, Water, and Fire. It will take about three minutes (to let the cortical brain know they won't be here for an hour), so let's begin.

We begin with the first element, Earth, which is grounding, calm, secure, at ease in the present moment. Take a moment or two to "land' here, to be here now.

Please place both feet on the ground and feel where you are seated supporting you.

Look around and notice three new things. What do you see, what do you hear? Any smells? How about the temperature on your skin?

The second element is Air, and we focus on the breath, which is centering.

Notice the breath going in gently through the nose, gently out through the mouth. We want the breath to have longer exhales, shorter inhales through the nose, to engage the relaxation response.

The third element is Water. Notice the Water in your mouth, which is called saliva. Sometimes when we are stressed the mouth dries out. So, make the mouth moister (and also let the brain know you are not in danger) by moving the tongue around to create moisture.

The fourth element is Fire. Now please close your eyes (if you are comfortable doing so, otherwise just soften the gaze). And now with the Fire element, we are going to light up the imagination to bring into our mind a place where we have been before. Notice the colors that are there, the sounds that you hear, the temperature on your skin.

Optional: Now in your calm, comfortable place, let's bring in your own tribe— your IRS (the inner team you can count on when you need some support). These are real or imagined, two- or four-legged, or maybe a winged being. For example:

- A wise figure, which can be a religious figure, such as God or Jesus, or a parent, teacher, sponsor, therapist, etc.

- A Protector figure, such as a power animal, superhero, or God.

- A Comforter, which may be a parent, God, a pet, an angel, a friend, a grandparent.

- A "fun" being, such as a best friend, memory of a fun time, super hero, rock star, maybe children, to remind you to lighten up when you are taking things way too seriously.

Now let's tap this in, so you call on them when you need.

The belief they reported feeling after, such as, "I can do this," "I am smart," "My life is limitless," "Taking the time to relax is important," "I want to have a full life without drugs and alcohol," "It is ok to ask for help," "Relaxation helps, I need help."

When you are ready to come back to the present moment, just breathe out through your mouth slowly and open your eyes. Notice how you feel now.

Tapping points: The Emotional Freedom Technique (EFT)

EFT is a simple and effective form of meridian energy therapy. Some call it "emotional acupuncture" but without the needles. You may have heard of it, and it looks weird. The good news is...it works!

We will be tapping with our fingertips on certain key power points (meridians/acupressure points) on the body. While tapping, we will feel and notice the sensation in the body or see the image/belief in the mind that needs to be released. Tap on the meridian points while making a statement of release and simultaneously state a healing affirmation to reprogram the habitual thoughts and beliefs: I release and let go... I choose...

Gary Craig created EFT in 1995. He says try it on everything!

Light Stream

This exercise (revised by Shafer in 2023) can be used to shut down an incomplete session, or instead of the Container exercise (see Chapter 8 and above).

Please allow your eyes to close or soften your gaze. Notice your whole body in this room, in this moment, and be aware of the great work you did today in this session. Acknowledge the courage you have to do the work.

Now please place your hands palms up or down on your thighs, so they are not touching, and both feet on the ground. (Pause.)

Now that you have shut your eyes or softened your gaze, we are going to enter the world of imagination—and everybody has one—where anything and everything can happen. There is no right way or wrong way to do this exercise, only your way.

Bring your focus to the bottom of your feet. And on the bottom of your feet is a trap door. See, sense, and feel this trap door open and out flows a beautiful, healing color of light. When you see this color of healing light, tell me what color it is. (Pause.)

See, sense, and feel this beautiful, healing color of [say the color out loud], and see, sense, and feel it flow out of the bottom of your feet, making its way up your body, swirling around the ankles, calves, around the knees, hips, tail bone, groin, stomach, rib cage, lungs, heart, shoulders, down both arms, to the hands and the fingers, including the finger tips, then back up the arms to the shoulders, neck, jaw, face, around both ears, the space between the ears, the forehead, around your brain, to the top of the head.

Then oops—there is another trap door and it opens. Again, see, sense, and feel this beautiful healing color of [say the color again here], flowing out of the top of your head. Now feel this healing light flow back down your body, flowing down like an umbrella or halo of energy surrounding you on all sides. The front of the body, sides of the body, back of the body, all surrounding your whole body like a cocoon as is continues to flow down and meet where it is flowing out of the trap door on the bottom of your feet.

Now enjoy the sensation of this healing [say the color out loud again here] light all around you. (Pause.)

And without moving your hands or feet, keeping the eyes closed, how do you feel?

Please note: Hopefully, the client will say something like, "calm", "peaceful," "at ease." If the client says something like, "Nothing's changed" or "I am sad," they may need to review their blocking beliefs at the next session. But for now, have them focus on a part of the body that is really enjoying this sensation of the healing light and WAIT.

The therapist continues with, "When you feel ready to come back to this moment and complete the session for today, take a long, slow exhale out through the mouth and open your eyes."

Then only ask: "How do you feel now?" This is how you will know if the exercise "took." Do not engage in discussion. Just remind them that the brain will continue to ponder and be curious about what went on today. You can tell them to take notes or write down any dreams they may have to discuss in the next session.

Spiral Technique

This exercise was adapted from Elan Shapiro (2012). Close your eyes and as you enter the world of imagination. Try to get an image or situation in your mind of something that is bothering you right now at about a 3 on a scale of 0–10, where 0 is neutral or nothing and 10 is as bad as it can get.

As you think about this, scan your body and notice where you are holding this disturbance. It may be in your head, stomach, neck, chest, shoulders, back. It may be in one place or several.

Now pretend that feeling or sensation is "energy" moving like a spiral. Which direction is your spiral of energy moving? Clockwise or counterclockwise? Take a few moments to concentrate on the feeling in your body for a few moments.

Now in your imagination, see yourself gently change the direction of the spiral in your body. For instance, if it was originally clockwise, gently change it to counterclockwise.

Notice what happens to the sensations in your body now.

If the shift feels better (calming, soothing, etc.), take a long, slow, and deep breath and tap in any enhancing sensations you have now. Enjoy this sensation. When you are ready, lower your hands, and breathe out and open your eyes.

Please note: When your client opens their eyes, ask, "How do you feel?" If one direction or the change of direction does not feel better or lessen the disturbance, or nothing happens, try another exercise.

Releasing Anxiety: Blue Light

The intention of this exercise (adapted from Epstein 1989) is to stop worrying or making up stories about the future and to release the anxiety.

Close your eyes and breathe out three long, slow breaths.

Now see yourself entering a beautiful meadow on a beautiful day. See yourself taking in the blue-golden light, a mixture of the warm (not hot), bright, golden sun, and the cloudless, blue sky, and breathing out carbon dioxide as gray smoke, which you watch drift away and disappear.

Let the blue light circulate through your blood stream, reaching everywhere in your being, helping you to feel calmer and quiet. Let the blue light circulate through your fingers and beyond, to circle around your whole body in a blue sapphire glow.

See, sense, and feel the inner and outer blue light linking. Know that your whole body is a bridge allowing this linking. When you see the blue light link, know the anxiety has passed.

Then breathe out through the mouth slowly and open your eyes.

Settling-In Exercise for Groups

Allow yourself to land here in this moment and place. Acknowledge yourself for choosing to come to this group tonight to take care of you.

Now notice the direction you are facing. Like the points of a compass, are you facing the direction the sun rises or the sun sets, or maybe to the north or south. Just allow yourself to get oriented to the direction you are facing.

And now notice the pull of gravity. Let it help you land and remain here on the Earth beneath you, feeling supported and held by the Earth beneath you, steady, solid, grounded.

Now be aware of your whole body, the position of the head, the trunk of your body, the arms, legs.

Now be aware of the room around you, the walls, the ceiling, the floor. Sense the space around you and the place you occupy in it.

Sense and notice the sensations you are aware of around you, such as sounds, the temperature of the air on your skin, smells, and any sensations you feel in the body.

Now bring your attention and focus to the place behind the eyelids and notice the light you see there.

Notice what you are sensing in your body now, the space you are occupying in your body, in this room, and within this group.

As you contemplate this, think about what is capturing your mind at this moment and what you would like to share with this group, maybe what you learned about yourself recently, and what you want to focus on now.

When you are ready, taking your time, breathe out slowly three times and open your eyes.

Go-To Resources and Bibliography

Go-to resources

These resources for expanding your falling awake journey include places, teachers, and bodies of work that may be of interest:

Places and teachers

Amrit Yoga Institute, Salt Springs, FL: https://amrityoga.org

Angela Farmer, co-founder of Omega Institute for Holistic Studies, Rhinebeck, New York: www.eomega. org and https://kripalu.org/resources/angela-farmer-yoga-activism-and-reconnecting-body

Brainspotting International, for all the latest research, trainings offered, information and how to find a Brainspotting therapist: https://brainspotting.com/international

EMDRIA (EMDR International Association), for all the latest research, trainings offered, information and how to find an EMDR therapist by zip code: www.emdria.org

Essence, Mind-Body Studio, Diana Spiess, Maumee, OH: www.dianaspiess.net

The FUN® Program with Dr. Kathy Shafer: https://limitlesspotentials.com/fun-program and Yoga Nidra Network: www.yoganidranetwork.org (including free downloads)

Himalayan Institute, Honesdale, PA: https://himalayaninstitute.org

I AM Yoga Nidra® with Dr. Kamini Desai (also an app): https://iameducation.org

Insight Yoga with Sarah and Ty Powers: www.sarahandtypowers.com

International Association of Yoga Therapists: www.iayt.org

Jennifer Reis, Creator of Divine Sleep® Yoga Nidra: www.JenniferReissYoga.com

John Vosler, multi-lineage Yoga Nidra educator: www.johnvosler.com

Julie Lusk, Wholesome Resources: https://wholesomeresources.com

Kripalu Center for Yoga & Health, Lenox, MA: https://kripalu.org

LifeForce Yoga® Training with Amy Weintraub (author of *Yoga for Depression*): www.amyweingraub. com/lifeforce-yoga

Mindfulness meditation with Jon Kabat-Zinn, PhD: www.mindful.org/everyday-mindfulness-with-jon-kabat-zinn

Sivananda Ashram Yoga Retreat, Bahamas: https://sivandabahamas.org

Yoga of Recovery® with Durga Leela, Yoga and the 12-Step approach: https://yogaofrecovery.com

Bodies of work and videos

Animated Rat Park: www.youtube.com/watch?v=xNmEboNEnd8

Bob Newhart, Just Stop It: www.youtube.com/watch?v=ZyT-coZycnk

Chalk Talk with Father Martin: www.youtube.com/watch?v=UzH6MfknWDo

Gabor Maté TED talk: Authenticity vs. Attachment: www.youtube.com/watch?v=l3bynimi8HQ

Gottman videos on how to save a marriage/relationship: www.youtube.com/watch?v=-Yujtw7CUJk

Just Breathe video: www.youtube.com/watch?v=-YEZnrySrtQ

Still Face Experiment: www.youtube.com/watch?v=YTTSXc6sARg

The Onion (satirical news): Lives Ruined by AA: www.theonion.com/aa-destroying-the-social-lives-of-thousands-of-once-fun-1819594912

The Lost Weekend, 1945 American drama film noir directed by Billy Wilder, and starring Ray Milland and Jane Wyman. It was based on Charles R. Jackson's 1944 novel of the same name about an alcoholic writer

Uprooting Addiction: Healing from the Ground Up, film by Hope Payson: https://hopepayson.com/documentary

Bibliography

Abel, N. and O'Brien, J. (2015) *Treating Addictions with EMDR Therapy and the Stages of Change.* New York: Springer Publishing.

Andrade, J., Kavanagh, D., and Baddeley, A. (1997) "Eye movements reduce image vividness and emotionality." *The British Journal of Clinical Psychology* 39, 209–223.

APA (American Psychiatric Association) (2013) *Diagnostic and Statistical Manual of Mental Disorders (5th Edition).* Arlington, VA: American Psychiatric Association.

April, E. (2021) *You're Not Dying: You're Just Waking Up.* [Independently published.]

Arora, I. (2015) *Mudra: The Sacred Secret.* Minneapolis, MN: Yog Sadhna.

Arora, I. (2019) *Yoga: Ancient Heritage, Tomorrow's* Vision. Minneapolis, MN: Yog Sadhna.

Badenoch, B. (2008) *Being a Brain-Wise Therapist: A Practical Guide to Interpersonal Neurobiology* (Norton Series on Interpersonal Neurobiology). Illustrated edition. New York: W.W. Norton & Co.

Badenoch, B, (2011) *The Brain-Savvy Therapists Workbook: A Companion to Being a Brain-Wise Therapist.* New York: W.W. Norton & Co.

Badenoch, B, (2018) *The Heart of Trauma: Healing the Embodied Brain in the Context of Relationships.* New York: W.W. Norton & Co.

Bae, H. and Kim, D. (2012) "Desensitization of triggers and urge reprocessing for an adolescent with internet addiction disorder." *Journal of EMDR Practice and Research* 6, 2, 73–81.

Barker, M. (2024) "Ready or not, AI is here." *Psychotherapy Networker,* January/February. www.psychotherapynetworker.org/article/ready-or-not-ai-is-here

Barrett, L. (2021) *Seven and a Half Lessons About the Brain.* New York: Mariner Books.

Baumann, M. (2020) *Brainspotting with Children and Adolescents: An Attuned Treatment Approach for Effective Brain-Body Healing.* Vienna: Monika Baumann Publisher.

Beltrán-Carrillo, J., Mejias, A., González-Cutre, D., and Jiménez-Loaisa, A. (2022) "Elements behind sedentary lifestyles and unhealthy eating habits in individuals with severe obesity." *International Journal of Qualitative Studies in Health and Well-being* 17, 1, 2056967. doi: 10.1080/17482631.2022.2056967.

Benson, H. (1975) *The Relaxation Response.* New York: HarperCollins.

Berceli, D. (2005) *Trauma Releasing Exercises (TRE): A Revolutionary New Method for Stress/Trauma Recovery.* North Charleston, SC: BookSurge, LLC.

Berg, I. (1994) *Family Based Services: A Solution-Focused Approach.* New York: W.W. Norton & Co.

Bergner, D. (2022) "Open minds: A new movement asks whether people with severe mental conditions should accept the voices in their heads—Rather than suppress them with medication." *The New York Times Magazine,* May 22, 44–53.

Bermann, U. (2012) "Consciousness examined: An introduction to the foundations of neurobiology for EMDR." *Journal of EMDR Practice and Research* 6, 3, 87–91.

Bernstein, G. (2016) *The Universe Has Your Back: Transform Fear to Faith.* Vista, CA: Hay House.

Black, C. (1993) *Changing Course: Healing From Loss, Abandonment, and Fear.* Minnesota, MN: Hazelden.

Blum, D. (2022) "'One foot in the present, one foot in the past:' Understanding EMDR. The once-experimental trauma treatment has become increasingly popular. Here's how the therapy works." *The New York Times,* September 19. www.nytimes.com/2022/09/19/well/emdr-therapy.html on 3/30/23

Brondani, M., Alan, R., and Donnelly, L. (2017) "Stigma of addiction and mental illness in healthcare: The case of patients' experiences in dental settings." *PLoS ONE* May 22. doi: 10.1371/journal.pone.0177388.

Brown, B. (2015) *Rising Strong: The Reckoning, The Rumble, The Revolution*. New York: Random House.

Brown, B. (2018) *Dare to Lead: Brave Work. Tough Conversations. Whole Hearts*. New York: Random House.

Brown, S., Gilman, S., Goodman, E., Adler-Tapie, R., and Freng, S. (2015) "Integrating trauma treatment in drug court: Combining EMDR therapy and seeking safety." *Journal of EMDR Practice and Research 9*, 3, 125–136.

Browning, C. (1999) "Floatback and floatforward: Techniques for linking past, present and future." *EMDRIA Newsletter 4*, 3, 12, 34.

Carr, D. (2023) "Tell me why it hurts: How Bessel van der Kolk's once controversial theory of trauma became the dominate way we make sense of our lives." *New York Magazine*, July 31.

Carson, R.D. (1983) *Taming Your Gremlin: A Guide to Enjoying Yourself*. New York: Quill.

CDC (Centers for Disease Control and Prevention) (2020) "Infographic: 6 guiding principles to a trauma-informed approach." www.cdc.gov/orr/infographics/6_principles_trauma_info.htm

Cheever, S. (2015) *Drinking in America: Our Secret History*. New York: Twelve Hatchette Book Group.

Chödrön, P. (2010) *Taking the Leap: Freeing Ourselves from Old Fears and Habits*. Boulder, CO: Shambhala Publications.

Chödrön, P. (2022) *How We Live Is How We Die*. Boulder, CO: Shambhala Publications.

Chopich, E.J. and Paul, M. (1990) *Healing Your Aloneness: Finding Wholeness Through Your Inner Child*. New York: Harper & Row.

Choudhury, B. (1978) *Bikram's Beginning Yoga Class*. New York: Tarcher.

Christman, S.D., Garvey, K.J., Propper, R.E., and Phaneuf, K.A. (2003) "Bilateral eye movements enhance the retrieval of episodic memories." *Neuropsychology 17*, 2, 221–229.

Conti, P. (2023) *Trauma: The Invisible Epidemic. How Trauma Works and How We Can Heal from It*. Boulder, CO: Sounds True.

Cope, S. (2006) *The Wisdom of Yoga: A Seeker's Guide to Extraordinary Living*. New York: Bantam Books.

Cori, J.L. (2010) *The Emotionally Absent Mother: A Guide to Self-Healing and Getting the Love You Missed*. New York: The Experiment.

Corn, S. (2019) *Revolution of the Soul: Awaken to Love Through Raw Truth, Radical Healing, and Conscious Action*. Boulder, CO: Sounds True.

Corrigan, F. and Christie-Sands, J. (2020) "An innate brainstem self-other system involving orienting, affective, and polyvalent relational seeking: Some clinical implications for a 'deep brain reorienting' trauma psychotherapy approach." *Medical Hypothesis 136*, 10952, 1–10.

Corrigan, F. and Grand, D. (2013) "Brainspotting: Recruiting the midbrain for accessing and healing sensorimotor memories of traumatic activation." *Medical Hypothesis 80*, 759–766.

Corrigan, F., Fisher, J.J., and Nutt, D. (2011) "Breaking free: A mind-body approach to retraining the brain." *Psychotherapy Networker*, March.

Craig, G. ([1995] 2008) *The Emotional Freedom Technique Manual*. Toronto, ON: Energy Psychology Press.

D'Antoni, F., Matiz, A., Fabbro, F., and Cresentini, C. (2022) "Psychotherapeutic techniques for distressing memories: A comparative study between EMDR, brainspotting, and body scan meditation." *International Journal of Environmental Research and Public Health 19*, 1142, 1–16.

Damasio, A. (1999) *The Feeling of What Happens: Body and Emotion in the Making of Consciousness*. New York: Harcourt College Publishers.

Dana, D. (2018) *The Polyvagal Theory in Therapy: Engaging the Rhythm of Regulation*. New York: W.W. Norton & Co.

Dana, D. (2021) *Anchored: How to Befriend Your Nervous System Using Polyvagal Theory*. Boulder, CO: Sounds True.

Dansinger, S. (2019) "EMDR therapy and addiction: The new frontier." *Counselor Magazine*, March 4, 28–32.

de Shazer, S. and Dolan, Y. (2007) *More Than Miracles: The State of the Art of Solution-Focused Brief Therapy*. New York: Routledge.

Del Monte, D. (2023) "Brain, trauma, and psychotherapy: A neurobiological view on EMDR." Presentation at the EMDR Canada Annual Virtual Conference, April 23 [Live webinar].

Desai, K. (2017) *Yoga Nidra: The Art of Transformational Sleep.* Silver Lake, WI: Lotus Press.

Dinsmore-Tuli, U. (2014) *Yoni Shakti: A Woman's Guide to Power and Freedom Through Yoga and Tantra.* London: YogaWords.

Dinsmore-Tuli, U. and Tuli, N. (2022) *Yoga Nidra Made Easy: Deep Relaxation to Improve Sleep, Relieve Stress, and Boost Energy and Creativity.* London: Hay House UK.

Doidge, N. (2007) *The Brain that Changes Itself: Stories of Personal Triumph from the Frontiers of Brain Science.* New York: Penguin Books.

Doidge, N. (2016) *The Brain's Way of Healing: Remarkable Discoveries and Recoveries from the Frontier of Neuroplasticity.* New York: Penguin Books.

Dominguez, S. (2022) "EMDR therapy for depression: Implications for mental health." *Go With That Magazine,* Winter, 27, 1, 5–10.

Dore, J. (2021) *Tarot for Change: Using the Cards for Self-Care, Acceptance, and Growth.* New York: Random House.

Douillard, J. (1994) *Body, Mind, and Sport: The Mind-Body Guide to Lifelong Fitness and Your Personal Best.* New York: Crown Publishing.

Eden, D. (2008) *Energy Medicine for Women: Aligning Your Body's Energies to Boost Your Health and Vitality.* New York: Penguin Books.

Emerson, D. (2015) *Trauma-Sensitive Yoga in Therapy: Bringing the Body into Treatment.* New York: W.W. Norton & Co.

Engelhard, I.M., van den Hout, M.A., Janssen, W.C., and van der Beek, J. (2010) "Eye movements reduce vividness and emotionality of 'flashforwards'." *Behavior Research and Therapy* 48, 5, 442–447.

Epstein, G. (1989) *Healing Visualizations: Creating Health Through Imagery.* New York: Bantam Books.

Epstein, G. (1994) *Healing into Immortality: A New Spiritual Medicine of Healing Stories and Imagery.* New York: Bantam Books.

Epstein, G. and Fedoroff, B. (eds) (2012) *The Encyclopedia of Mental Imagery.* New York: ACMI Press.

Felitti, V.J., Anda, R.F., Nordenberg, D., Williamson, D.F., *et al.* (1998) "Relationship of childhood abuse and household dysfunction to many of the leading causes of death in adults: The Adverse Childhood Experiences (ACE) Study." *American Journal of Preventive Medicine* 14, 4, 245–258.

Folan, L. (2005) *Lilias! Yoga Gets Better with Age.* Emmaus, PA: Rodale Books.

Forbes, B. (2011) *Yoga for Emotional Balance: Simple Practices to Help Relieve Anxiety and Depression.* Boulder, CO: Shambhala Publications, Inc.

Forgash, C. and Copeley, M. (2008) *Healing the Heart of Trauma and Dissociation with EMDR and Ego State Therapy.* New York: Springer Publishing.

Fraser, G. (1991) "The dissociation table technique: A strategy for working with ego-state therapy." *Dissociation* 4, 4, 205–213.

Frausin, A. and Grinder, J. (2017) "Real origins of EMDR (eye movement desensitization and reprocessing): The genius behind EMDR reveals the true story." https://mindmaster.ro/Portals/0/Historie_EMDR_Wingwave.pdf

Fridman, E. (2019) "Insecure attachment and drug misuse among women." *Journal of Social Work Practice in the Addictions* 19, 3, 223–237. https://doi.org/10.1080/1533256x.2019.1637229

Gannon. S. (2018) *The Magic Ten and Beyond: Daily Spiritual Practice for Greater Peace and Well Being.* New York: TarcherPerigree.

Gannon, S. and Life, D. (2002) *Jivamukti Yoga: Discover the Unique Energy and Spirit of the Yoga that Can Transform Your Life!* New York: Ballantine Books.

Gard, T., Noggle, J., Park, C., Vago, D., and Wilson, A. (2014) "Potential self-regulatory mechanisms of yoga for psychological health." *Frontiers in Human Neuroscience.* doi:10.3389/fnhum2014.00770.

Gawain, S. (1978) *Creative Visualization.* Berkeley, CA: New World Library.

Gendlin, E.T. (1982) *Focusing.* New York: Bantam Books.

Gonzalez, A. and Mosquera, D. (2012) *EMDR and Dissociation: The Progressive Approach.* AbeBooks

Grand, D. (2001) *Emotional Healing at Warp Speed: The Power of EMDR.* New York: Harmony Books.

Grand, D. (2013) *Brainspotting: The Revolutionary New Therapy for Rapid and Effective Change.* Boulder, CO: Sounds True.

Grand, D. (2021) "Brainspotting as a Neuroexperiential Process for Healing and Expansion." Keynote Address at the 2ndd International Brainspotting Conference, July, Denver, Colorado.

Grand, D. and Goldberg, A. (2011) *This Is Your Brain on Sports: Beating Blocks, Slumps, and Performance Anxiety for Good!* New York: Competitive Advantage.

Grossman, D. and Christensen, L. (2004) *On Combat: The Psychology and Physiology of Deadly Conflict in War and Peace.* New York: Open Road Media.

Gurda, K. (2015) "Critical analysis and discussion of three novel approaches." *Journal of Aggression, Maltreatment, and Trauma 24, 7, 773–793.*

Hanson Lasater, J. and Lasater, I.K. (2009) *What We Say Matters: Practicing Nonviolent Communication.* Boulder, CO: Shambhala.

Hase, M., Schallmayer, S., and Sack, M. (2008) "EMDR reprocessing of the addiction memory: Pretreatment, posttreatment, and 1-month follow-up." *Journal of EMDR Practice and Research* 2, 3, 170–179.

Hately Aldous, S. (2007) *Therapeutic Yoga for the Shoulders and Hips.* Calgary, AB: Functional Synergy.

Hawkins, D. (2012) *Letting Go: The Pathway of Surrender.* London: Hay House UK.

Hensley, B. (2016) *An EMDR Therapy Primer: From Practicum to Practice.* Second edition. New York: Springer Publishing.

Horowitz, M., Wilner, N., and Alvarez, W. (1979) "Impact of Event Scale: A measure of subjective stress." *Psychosomatic Medicine 41, 3, 209–218.*

Horton, L., Schwartzberg, C., Goldberg, C., Grieve, F., and Brdecka, L. (2024) "Brainspotting: A treatment for posttraumatic stress disorder." *International Body Psychotherapy Journal 1, 22,* 57–69. https://ibpj.org/issues/articles/Horton,%20Schwartzberg,%20Goldberg,%20Grieve,%20Brdecka%20-%20Brainspotting.pdf

Jacobson, E. (1962) *You Must Relax: Practical Methods for Reducing Tensions of Modern Living* (5th edn.). New York: McGraw-Hill.

Jarero, I. (2023) "Fire in the belly: The history of the butterfly hug, the EMDR-IGTP, and the ASSYST-Treatment Procedures." *Go With That Magazine,* Summer, 28, 3, 2–10.

Jordan, J.A. (2019) "Alcoholics Anonymous: A vehicle for achieving capacity for secure attachment relationships and adaptive affect regulation." *Journal of Social Work Practice in the Addictions* 19, 1, 1–22. https://doi.org/10.1080/1533256x.2019.1638180

Judith, A. (2015) *Chakra Yoga.* Woodbury, MN: Llewllyn Productions.

Kabat-Zinn, J. (1994) *Wherever You Go, There You Are: Mindfulness Meditation in Everyday Life.* New York: Hyperion.

Kabat-Zinn, J. (2018) *Falling Awake: How to Practice Mindfulness in Everyday Life.* New York: Hachette Books.

Kaelen, M. (2017) "The Psychological and Human Brain Effects of Music in Combination with Psychedelic Drugs." PhD Dissertation, Imperial College, London.

Kaminoff, L. and Matthews, A. (2011) *Yoga Anatomy* (Second edn.). Abingdon: Human Kinetics.

Kase, R. (2023) *Polyvagal-Informed EMDR: A Neurological Approach to Healing.* New York: W.W. Norton & Co.

Keenan, P., Farrell, D., Keenan, L., and Ingham, C. (2018) "Compulsive Disorder (OCD) using Eye Movement Desensitization and Reprocessing (EMDR) therapy: An ethno-phenomenological case series." *International Journal of Psychotherapy 22, 3, 74–91.*

Khalsa, M. (2008) *Meditations for Addictive Behavior: A System of Yogic Science with Nutritional Formulas.* Minneapolis, MN: Itasca Books.

Kiessling, R. (2005) "Integrating Resource Development Strategies into Your EMDR Practice." In R. Shapiro (ed.) *EMDR Solutions: Pathways to Healing* (pp.57–87). New York: W.W. Norton & Co.

Kiessling, R. (2021) *Intensive Training Manual.* www.scribd.com/document/558649578/EMDR-Training-Manual-249pags

Knipe, J. (1998) "The Blocking Beliefs Questionnaire." *EMDRIA Newsletter 7, 4, 5–6.* Winter.

Knipe, J. (2009) "Shame is My Safe Place: Adaptive Information Processing Methods of Resolving Chronic Shame-Based Depression." In R. Shapiro (ed.) *EMDR Solutions II: For Depression, Eating Disorders, and More* (pp.49–89). New York: Norton.

Knipe, J. (2019) *EMDR Toolbox: Theory and Treatment of Complex PTSD and Dissociation.* Second edition. New York: Springer.

Korn, D., and Leeds, A. (2002) "Preliminary evidence of efficacy for EMDR resource and development and installation in the stabilization of treatment of complex posttraumatic stress disorder." *Journal of Clinical Psychology* 58, 12, 1465–1487.

La Barre, D. (2010) *Issues in Your Tissues: Heal Body and Emotion from the Inside Out.* Haiku, HI: Healing Catalyst Press.

Lad, V. (2009) *Ayurveda: The Science of Self-Healing.* Silver Lake, WI: Lotus Press.

Lasater, J.H. (2007) *Relax and Renew: Restful Yoga for Stressful Times.* Berkeley, CA: Rodmell Press.

Lee, I. (2020) *Body and Brain Yoga Tai Chi.* Mesa, AZ: Best Life Media.

Leeds. A. (2016) *A Guide to the Standard EMDR Therapy Protocols for Clinicians, Supervisors, and Consultants.* New York: Springer Publishing.

Leeds, A.M. (2022) "The Positive Affect Tolerance and Integration protocol: A novel application of EMDR therapy procedures to help survivors of early emotional neglect learn to tolerate and assimilate moments of appreciation, praise, and affection." *Journal of EMDR Practice and Research* 16, 4, 202–214.

Leeds, A.M. (2023a) "An update on the progress and future of EMDR Therapy." EMDRAA 2023 Conference, May 5–7. https://vimeo.com/830101565

Leeds, A.M. (2023b) "Foundations of the positive affect tolerance protocol: The central role of interpersonal positive affect regulation in attachment and self-regulation." *Journal of EMDR Practice and Research*, 17, 3, 1–20.

Leela, D. (2022) *Yoga of Recovery: Integrating Yoga an Ayurveda with Modern Recovery Tools for Addiction.* Philadelphia, PA: Singing Dragon.

Levine, P. (1997) *Waking the Tiger: Healing Trauma.* Berkeley, CA: North Atlantic Books.

Levine, P. (2005) *Healing Trauma: A Pioneering Program for Restoring the Wisdom of Your Body.* Boulder, CO: Sounds True.

LeWine, H. (2024) "Understanding the stress response: Chronic activation of this survival mechanism impacts health." Harvard Health Publishing, 3 April. www.health.harvard.edu/staying-healthy/understanding-the-stress-response

Lind-Kyle, P. (2010). *Heal Your Mind, Rewire Your Brain: Applying the Exciting New Science of Brain Synchrony for Creativity, Peace and Prescence.* Toronto, ON: Energy Psychology Press.

Liu, K., Chen, Y., Wu, D., Lin, R., Wang, Z., and Pan, L. (2020) "Effects of progressive relaxation on anxiety and deep sleep quality in patients with COVID-19." *Complementary Therapies in Clinical Practice* 39,1–4.

Lobel, T. (2014) *Sensation: The New Science of Physical Intelligence.* New York: Aytria Books.

Long, R. (2005) *The Key Muscles of Hatha Yoga: Scientific Keys Volume I.* Bandha Yoga Publishers.

Long, R. (2008) *The Key Poses of Hatha Yoga: Your Guide to Functional Anatomy in Yoga.* Bandha Yoga Publishers.

Luber, M. (2010) *Eye Movement Desensitization and Reprocessing (EMDR) Scripted Protocols.* Springer Publishing.

Lusk, J. (2021) *Yoga Nidra Meditations: 24 Scripts for True Relaxation.* Minnesota, MN: Llewellyn.

Lutz, J. (2021) *Trauma Healing in the Yoga Zone: A Guide for Mental Health Professionals, Yoga Therapists, and Teachers.* London: Handspring Publishing.

Manfield, P., Lovett, J., Engel, L., and Manfield, D. (2017) "Use of the flash technique in EMDR Therapy: Four case examples." *Journal of EMDR Practice and Research* 11, 4, 195–205.

Marich, J. (2011) *EMDR Made Simple: 4 Approaches to Using EMDR with Every Client.* Eau Claire, WI: Premier Publishing & Media.

Marich, J. (2012) *Trauma and the Twelve Steps: A Complete Guide for Recovery.* Cornersburg, OH: Cornersburg Media.

Marich, J. (2023) *Dissociation Made Simple: A Stigma-Free Guide to Embracing Your Dissociative Mind and Navigating Daily Life.* Berkeley, CA: North Atlantic Books.

Marich, J. and Dansinger, S. (2018) *EMDR Therapy and Mindfulness for Trauma-Focused Care.* New York: Springer.

Marich, J. and Dansinger, S. (2022) *Healing Addiction with EMDR Therapy: A Trauma-Focused Guide.* New York: Springer.

Mason, H. and Birch, K. (eds) (2018) *Yoga for Mental Health.* London: Handspring Publishing.

Maté, G. (2022) *The Myth of Normal: Trauma, Illness, and Healing in a Toxic Culture.* New York: Avery.

Matthijssen, S., Browers, T., van Roozendaal, C., and de Jongh, A. (2021) "The effect of EMDR versus EMDR 2.0 on emotionality and vividness of aversive memories in a non-clinical sample." *European Journal of Psychotraumatology* 12, 1, 1956793. https://doi.org/10.1080/20008198.2021.1956793

Maxfield, L., Melnyk, W.T., and Hayman, C.A.G. (2008) "A working memory explanation for the effects of eye movements in EMDR." *Journal of EMDR Practice and Research* 2, 4, 247–261. https://doi.org/10.1891/1933-3196.2.4.247

Méndez, M.Z., Nijdam, M.J., Ter Heide, F.J.J., van de Aa, N., and Olff, M. (2018) "A five-day inpatient EMDR treatment program for PTSD: Pilot study." *European Journal of Psychotraumatology* 9, 1, 1425575.

Menon, S. (2022) *The Brain Forest*. Yarraville, VIC: Onwards & Upwards Psychology.

Merzenich, M. (2013) *Soft-Wired: How the New Science of Brain Plasticity Can Change Your Life*. Nashville, TN: Parnassus Publishing.

Meyers, T. (2022) *Yin Yoga Therapy and Mental Health: An Integrated Approach*. London and Philadelphia, PA: Singing Dragon.

Miller, J. (2023) *Body by Breath: The Science and Practice of Physical and Emotional Resilience*. Las vegas, NV: Victory Belt Publishing.

Miller, R. (2010a) "The feeling-state theory of impulse-control disorders and the Impulse-Control Disorder Protocol." *Traumatology* 16, 3, 2–10. https://doi.org/10.1177/1534765610365912

Miller, R. (2010b) *Yoga Nidra: A Meditative Practice for Deep Relaxation and Healing*. Boulder, CO: Sounds True, Inc.

Miller, R. (2015) *The iRest Program for Healing PTSD: A Proven-Effective Approach to Using Yoga Nidra Meditation and Deep Relaxation Techniques to Overcome Trauma*. Oakland, CA: New Harbinger Publications.

Miller, T. and Hendrie, D. (2008) *Substance Abuse Prevention Dollars and Cents: A Cost-Benefit Analysis*. DHHS Pub. No. (SMA) 07-4298. Rockville, MD: Center for Substance Abuse Prevention, Substance Abuse and Mental Health Services Administration.

Mintie, D. and Staples, J. (2018) *Reclaiming Life after Trauma: Healing PTSD with Cognitive-Behavioral Therapy and Yoga*. Rochester, VT: Healing Arts Press.

Moore, S. (2019) *Practical Yoga Nidra: A 10 Step Method to Reduce Stress, Improve Sleep, and Restore Your Spirit*. Emeryville, CA: Rockridge Press.

Morandi, A. and Nambi, A. (eds) (2013) *An Integrated View of Health and Well Being: Bridging Indian and Western Knowledge*. Volume 5. New York: Springer.

Murray, K. (2011) "Container." *Journal of EMDR Practice and Research* 5, 1, 29–32. doi:10.1891/1933-3196.5.1.29.

Nelson, T. (ed.)(2010) *Doing Something Different: Solution-Focused Brief Therapy Practices*. New York: Routledge.

Nestor, J. (2020) *Breath: The New Science of a Lost Art*. New York: Riverhead Books.

Nielsen, J.A., Zielinski, B.A., Ferguson, M.A., Lainhart, J.E., and Anderson, J.S. (2013) "An evaluation of the left-brain vs. right-brain hypothesis with resting state functional connectivity Magnetic Resonance Imaging." *PLoS ONE* 8, e71275–11.

Panksepp, J. (1998) *Affective Neuroscience: The Foundation of Human and Animal Emotions*. New York: Oxford University Press.

Parnell, L. (2007) *A Therapist's Guide to EMDR: Tools and Techniques for Successful Treatment*. New York: W.W. Norton & Co.

Parnell, L. (2008) *Tapping In: A Step-By-Step Guide to Activating Your Healing Resources Through Bilateral Stimulation*. Boulder, CO: Sounds True.

Parnell, L. (2013) *Attachment-Focused EMDR: Healing Relational Trauma*. New York: W.W. Norton & Co.

Parnell, L. (2018) *Rewiring the Addicted Brain: An EMDR-Based Treatment Model for Overcoming Addictive Disorders*. San Rafael, CA: Green Tara Press.

Parker, S., Bharati, S.V., and Fernandez, M. (2013) "Defining yoga-nidra: Traditional accounts, physiological research, and future directions." *International Journal of Yoga Therapy* 23, 1, 11–16.

Paulsen, S. (2017) *When There Are No Words: Repairing Early Trauma and Neglect from the Attachment Period with EMDR Therapy*. Bainbridge Island, WA: Bainbridge Institute for Integrative Psychology.

Payson-Call, A. ([1891], 1920) *Power Through Repose: The Laws of Transmission: Getting What You Want Through Mastery of The Mind, Body and Will*. Boston, MA: Little, Brown & Company.

Pollan, M. (2018) *How to Change Your Mind: What the New Science of Psychedelics Teaches Us About Consciousness, Dying, Addiction, Depression, and Transcendence*. New York: Penguin Books.

Porges, S.W. (2017) *The Pocket Guide to The Polyvagal Theory: The Transformative Power of Feeling Safe*. New York: W.W. Norton & Co.

Porges, S.W. (2022) "Polyvagal theory: A science of safety." *Frontiers in Integrative Neuroscience 16*, 1–15. https://doi.org/10.3389/fnint.2022.871227

Porges, S.W., Doussard-Roosevelt, J.A., and Mait, A.K. (1994) "Vagal tone and the physiological regulation of emotion." *Monographs of the Society for Research in Child Development 59*, 2–3, 250–283. https://doi.org/10.2307/1166144

Prinster, T. (2014) *Yoga for Cancer: A Guide to Managing Side Effects, Boosting Immunity, and Improving Recovery for Cancer Survivors*. Rochester, VT: Healing Arts Press.

Pyles, L., Cosgrave, D.T., Gardner, E., Raheim, S., *et al.* (2021) "'Could we just breathe for 30 seconds?' Social worker experiences of holistic engagement practice training." *Social Work 66*, 4, 285–296.

Rama, S. (1978) *Living with the Himalayan Masters*. Honesdale, PA: Himalayan Institute.

Rama, S. (1996) *Path of Fire and Light: Advanced Practices of Yoga*. Honesdale, PA: Himalayan Institute.

Rankin, L. (2022) *Sacred Medicine: A Doctor's Quest to Unravel the Mysteries of Healing*. Boulder, CO: Sounds True, Inc.

Remen, R.N. (1996) *Kitchen Table Wisdom: Stories that Heal*. New York: Riverhead Books.

Rosen, T. (2014) *Recovery 2.0. Move Beyond Addiction and Upgrade Your Life*. St Vista, CA: Hay House.

Ryba, C. (2022) *Pelvic Yoga Therapy for the Whole Woman: A Professional Guide*. London: Singing Dragon.

Salvador, M. (2021) "Brainspotting, Attunement, and Prescence in the Therapeutic Relationship." In G. Wolfrum (Ed.) *The Power of Brainspotting: An International Anthology*. www.asanger.de

SAMHSA (Substance Abuse and Mental Health Services Administration) (2023. *Practical Guide for Implementing a Trauma-Informed Approach*. SAMHSA Publication No. PEP23-06-05-005. Rockville, MD: National Mental Health and Substance Use Policy Laboratory. Substance Abuse and Mental Health Services Administration. http://store.samhsa.gov

Saraswati, S. (1976) *Yoga Nidra*. Delhi: Thomson Press Limited.

Sarno, J.E. (1991) *Healing Back Pain: The Mind-Body Connection*. New York: Warner Books.

Satchidananda, S.S. (translator and commentator) (1978) "The Yoga Sutras of Patanjali 1.2." *Integral Yoga Publications*, p.3 www.iyiva.org

Satir, V. (1976) *Making Contact*. Millbrae, CA: Celestial Arts.

Schwartz, A. (2016) *The Complex PTSD Workbook: A Mind-Body Approach to Regaining Emotional Control & Becoming Whole*. Berkeley, CA: Althea Press.

Schwartz, A. (2022) *Therapeutic Yoga for Trauma Recovery: Applying Principles of Polyvagal Theory for Self Discovery, Embodied Healing, and Meaningful Change*. Eau Claire: WI: PESI.

Schwartz, A. and Maiberger, B. (2018) *EMDR Therapy and Somatic Psychology: Interventions to Enhance Embodiment in Trauma Treatment*. New York: W.W. Norton & Co.

Sciarrino, N., DeLucia, C., O'Brien, K., and McAdams, K. (2017) "Assessing the effectiveness of yoga as a complementary and alternative treatment for post-traumatic stress disorder: A review and synthesis." *Journal of Alternative and Complementary Medicine 23*, 10, 747–755.

Shafer, K. (2010) "'Disease Free': First Session Exercise." In T.S. Nelson (ed.) *Doing Something Different: Solution-Focused Brief Therapy Practices* (Chapter 8). New York: Routledge.

Shafer, K. and Greenfield, F. (2000) *Asthma Free in 21 Days: The Breakthrough Mindbody Healing Program*. New York: W.W. Norton & Co.

Shapiro, E. (2012) "The four elements of stress reduction." YouTube [video]. www.youtube.com/watch?v=4StCjYm8nuo

Shapiro, F. (1995) *Eye Movement Desensitization and Reprocessing: Basic Principles, Protocols and Procedures*. New York: Guilford Press.

Shapiro, F. (2001) *Eye Movement Desensitization and Reprocessing: Basic Principles, Protocols, and Procedures*. Second edition. New York: Guilford Press.

Shapiro, F. (2002) *EMDR as an Integrative Psychotherapy Approach: Experts of Diverse Orientations Explore the Paradigm Prism*. Washington, DC: American Psychological Association Press.

Shapiro, F. (2007) "EMDR, adaptive information processing, and case conceptualization." *Journal of EMDR Practice and Research* 1, 2, 68–87.

Shapiro, F. (2012) *Getting Past Your Past: Take Control of Your Life with Self-Help Techniques from EMDR Therapy*. New York: Rodale Press.

Shapiro, F and Forrest, M. (1997) *EMDR: The Breakthrough Therapy for Overcoming Anxiety, Stress, and Trauma*. New York: Basic Books.

Shapiro, F., Vogelman-Sine, S., and Sine, L. (1994) "Eye Movement Desensitization and Reprocessing: Treating trauma and substance abuse." *Journal of Psychoactive Drugs* 26, 4, 379–391.

Shapiro, R. (ed.) (2005) *EMDR Solutions: Pathways to Healing Vol. 1 & 2*. New York: W.W. Norton & Co.

Shapiro, R. (ed.) (2009) *EMDR Solutions II: For Depression, Eating Disorders, Performance, and More*. New York: W.W. Norton & Co.

Shapiro, R. (2016) *Easy Ego State Interventions: Strategies for Working with Parts*. New York: W.W. Norton & Co.

Shapiro, R. (2020) *Doing Psychotherapy: A Trauma-informed Approach*. New York: W.W. Norton & Co.

Shaw, B. (2009) *YogaFit®: The Program for a More Powerful, Flexible, and Defined Physique*. Champaign, IL: Human Kinetics.

Sheldon, B. and Sheldon, A. (2022) *Complex Integration of Multiple Brain Systems in Therapy*. New York: W.W. Norton & Co.

Shivapremananda, S. (1997) *Yoga for Stress Relief*. New York: Random House.

Siegel, D.J. (2002) "The Developing Mind and the Resolution of Trauma: Some Ideas About Information Processing and an Interpersonal Neurobiology of Psychotherapy." In F. Shapiro (Ed.) *EMDR as an Integrative Psychotherapy Approach: Experts of Diverse Origins Explore the Paradigm Prism* (pp.85–121). Washington, DC: American Psychological Association.

Siegel, D.J. (2013) *Brainstorm: The Power and Purpose of the Teenage Brain*. New York: Penguin/Random House.

Siegel, D.J. (2018) *Aware: The Science and Practice of Presence*. New York: Penguin Random House.

Siegel, D.J. (2023) *IntraConnected: MWE (Me +We) As the Integration of Self, Identity, and Belonging*. New York: W.W. Norton & Co.

Siegel, D.J. and Drulis, C. (2023) "An interpersonal neurobiology perspective on the mind and mental health: Personal, public, and planetary well-being." *Annals of General Psychiatry* 22, 1, 5.

Siegel, D.J. and Payne Bryson, T. (2015) *The Whole-Brain Child Workbook: Practical Exercises, Worksheets, and Activities to Nurture Developing Minds*. Eau Claire, WI: PESI.

Sivananda Yoga Vedanta Center (2018) *Practical Ayurveda*. New York: Penguin Random House.

Sovik, R. (2005) *Moving Inward: The Journey to Meditation*. Honesdale, PA: Himalayan Institute Press.

Spence, J. (2021) *Trauma-Informed Yoga: A Toolbox for Therapists*. Eau Claire, WI: PESI.

Springsteen, B. and Stern, H. (2022) "The Drive that Makes Bruce Springsteen." Interview with Howard Stern on MSNBC, November 23.

Steffen, P.R., Hedges, D., and Matheson, R. (2022) "The brain is adaptive not triune: How the brain responds to threat, challenge and change." *Frontiers in Psychiatry*. doi: 10.3389/fpsyt.2022.802606.

Stickgold, R. (2002) "EMDR: A putative neurobiological mechanism of action." *Journal of Clinical Psychology* 58, 1, 61–75.

Stryker, R. ([1977] 2012) *The Four Desires: Creating a Life of Purpose, Happiness, Prosperity, and Freedom*. Vista, CA: Hay House.

Tebb, S. (1995) "An aid to empowering: A caregiving well-being scale." *Health and Social Work* 20, 2, 87–92.

Tigunait, P.R. (1996) *The Power of Mantra & The Mystery of Initiation*. Honesdale, PA: Himalayan Institute.

Tigunait, P.R. (2001) *At The Eleventh Hour: The Biography of Swami Rami*. Honesdale, PA: Himalayan.

Tigunait, P.R. (2019) *Vishoka Meditation: The Yoga of Inner Radiance*. Honesdale, PA: Himalayan Institute.

Van Dam, A. (2022) "Why have millions of Americans moved to these countries instead?" *The Washington Post*, December 23. www.washingtonpost.com/business/2022/12/23/american-emigrants

van den Hout, M., Muris, P., Salemink, E., and Kindt, M. (2001) "Autobiographical memories become less vivid and emotional after eye movements." *The British Journal of Clinical Psychology* 40, 121–130. doi: 10.1348/014466501163571

van der Kolk, B. (2002) "Trauma and memory." *Psychiatry and Clinical Neurosciences* 52, S1, S52–S64.

van der Kolk, B. (2014) *The Body Keeps the Score: Brain, Mind, and Body in the Healing of Trauma.* New York: Viking.

Walker, M. (2017) *Why We Sleep: Unlocking the Power of Sleep and Dreams.* New York: Scribner.

Wanck, B. (2019) "Science backs 'alternative' holistic healing." *Counselor Magazine*, 22–27.

Weintraub, A. (2004) *Yoga for Depression.* New York: Broadway Books.

Weintraub, A. (2012) *Yoga Skills for Therapists: Effective Practices for Mood Management.* New York: W.W. Norton & Co.

Weintraub, A. (2021) *Yoga for Your Mood Deck: 52 Ways to Shift Depression and Anxiety.* Boulder, CO: Sounds True.

Weiss, D.S. (2007) "The Impact of Event Scale: Revised." In J.P. Wilson and C.S.-K. Tang (eds) *Cross-Cultural Assessment of Psychological Trauma and PTSD* (pp.219–238). Springer Science + Business Media. https://doi.org/10.1007/978-0-387-70990-1_10

Whitfield, C. (1989) *Healing the Child Within: Discovery and Recovery for Adult Children of Dysfunctional Families* . Pompano Beach, FL: Health Communications.

Whitlock Burton, K. (2022) "Yoga, CBT provide long-term improvements in insomnia, worry." Medscape, September 1. www.medscape.com/viewarticle/980100?form=fpf

Wikipedia contributors (2024) "If You're Going Through Hell (Before the Devil Even Knows)." *Wikipedia, The Free Encyclopedia*. Retrieved July 18, 2024, from https://en.wikipedia.org/w/index.php?title=If_You%27re_Going_Through_Hell_(Before_the_Devil_Even_Knows)&oldid=1225852408

Wolfrum, G. (ed.) (2021) *The Power of Brainspotting: An International Anthology.* Asanger Verlag.

Yarema, T., Rhoda, D., and Brannigan, J. (2006) *Eat-Taste-Heal: An Ayurvedic Cookbook for Modern Living.* Chicago, IL: Five Elements Press.

Young, J.E., Zangwill, W.M., and Behary, W.E. (2002) "Combining EMDR and Schema-Focused Therapy: The Whole May Be Greater than the Sum of the Parts." in F. Shapiro (ed.) *EMDR as an Integrative Psychotherapy Approach* (pp.181–208). Washington, DC: American Psychological Association.

Zuckweiler, B. (1998) *Living in the Postmastectomy Body: Learning to Live In and Love Your Body Again.* Tumwater, WA: Hartley & Marks, Inc.

Zweig, C. (2021) *The Inner Work of Age: Shifting from Role to Soul.* Rochester, VT: Park Street Press.